HEALTHY
HEART

MOSELEY ROAD INC.
International Rights and Packaging
22 Knollwood Avenue
Elmsford, NY 10523
www.moseleyroad.com

President Sean Moore
General manager Karen Prince
Production and art director Adam Moore
Project designer Lisa Purcell

Photography Naila Ruechel
www.nailaruechel.com

Printed in Canada

ISBN 978-1-62669-202-2

21 20 19 18 17   1 2 3 4 5

HEALTHY
HEART

STRENGTHEN AND PROTECT YOUR HEART

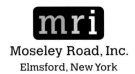

mri

Moseley Road, Inc.
Elmsford, New York

CONTENTS

A PLAN FOR HEALTH

The way to a healthy heart is healthy living, and the smartest plan for overcoming heart problems is, of course, preventing one from ever happening. The more healthy habits you introduce into your life, the more you reduce your risk of heart disease. And the benefits of a healthy heart are not just about living longer and looking and feeling great, good health can also have a positive influence on every aspect of your life.

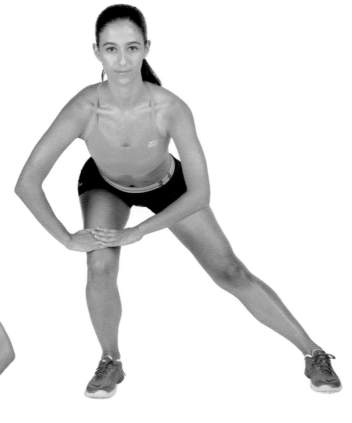

People today are increasingly aware of their personal levels of fitness—monitoring and recording their successes with tape measures, calipers, digital scales, diets and fitness apps, and activity trackers. And with good reason—the foods you eat and the amount of activity you choose to take part in can dramatically affect the overall health of your

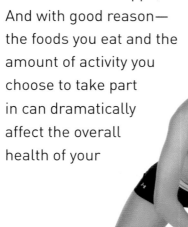

heart and the many other tissues that make up your cardiovascular system.

This book is a comprehensive guide to everything you'll need to know and do to sustain a healthy heart. As well offering advice on diet and lifestyle, it shows you how to get

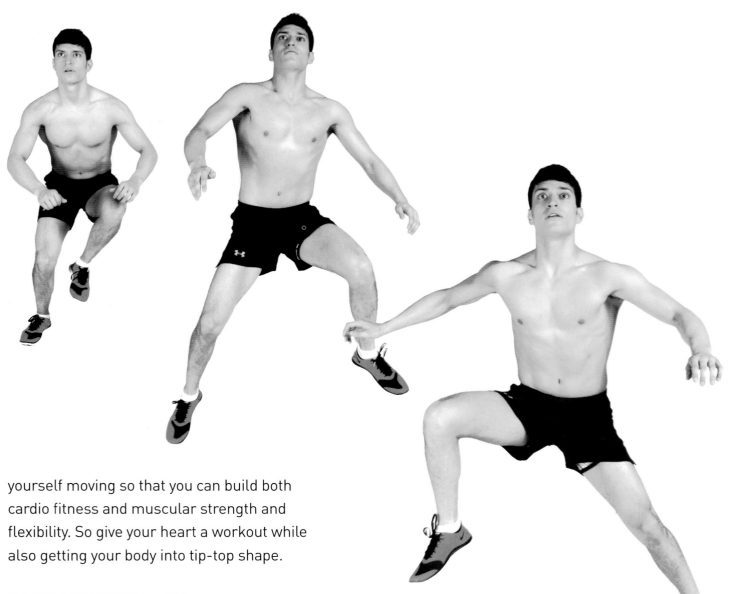

yourself moving so that you can build both cardio fitness and muscular strength and flexibility. So give your heart a workout while also getting your body into tip-top shape.

HOW TO USE THIS BOOK

The book is divided into two sections: Section One will help you to understand how your heart works and how to keep it healthy through smart choices. Section Two will take you through a series of workouts that can help you get your heart healthy—and to keep it that way.

The Healthy Heart workouts are divided into three levels of difficulty, and each level features two or three workouts. You'll find them listed on the first page of the level, which also includes a progress chart so that you can decide when to level up.

For each featured workout, you will see a rundown of the entire routine and a checklist that shows you what fitness equipment you'll need for that workout. Next, each exercise is shown in detail, with step-by-step instructions and photographs on how to perform it. You will also find an anatomical illustration that highlights the major muscles that the exercise targets. A handy at-a-glance guide lets you know what type of exercise it is (cardio, strength, or stretch), and any you'll need to gather.

SECTION ONE

TIPS FOR A HEALTHY HEART

Explore the many ways you can work toward getting your heart in shape, beginning with making changes to any part of your daily routine that detracts from that goal. In this section, you will find info on basic heart health, such as how to calculate your target heart rate, and some of the top tips for a Healthy Heart lifestyle.

LOVE YOUR HEART

The heart is often aptly described as the body's engine room, pumping blood via a truly vast network of arteries, veins, and capillaries, to continuously resupply the body with oxygen and vital nutrients, while washing away harmful waste matter. The food you eat, the activities you enjoy, and the stresses you endure can all dramatically effect the health of your heart. If you love life, you've simply got to love your heart. Here's how.

Given the heart's many essential functions, it only seems sensible to take care of it and by picking up Healthy Heart you have already made a great start. This book is your roadmap to gaining and sustaining a healthy heart using a broad range of exercises designed to build strength, stamina, and flexibility. But looking after your heart isn't all about exercise; you need to eat well, sleep well, work well and play well—most of the time! So, let's check out the road ahead ,bearing in mind that the safest and surest route is rarely the shortest, while remembering, too, that we want the journey itself to be fun right from the start, which is exactly how it should be. Once you set your heart on health, the journey itself gets better with every step. So, let's get started!

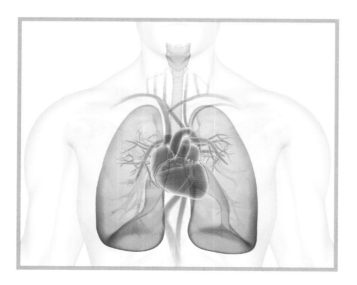

PLAN FOR A HEALTHY HEART

Ben Franklin famously said that "if you fail to plan, you are planning to fail." Although truly one of the greatest of the great, Franklin himself failed to plan for good health and suffered from chronic obesity and gout in later life. In his autobiography, Franklin listed 13 virtues, the first of which was "Temperance: Eat not to dullness, drink not to elevation." He was the first to admit that he often fell short of his own ideals, but we can learn from his failures just as much as we can learn from his countless successes, and, like him, we can and should cut ourselves some slack. If we slip up now and again, we pick ourselves up, dust ourselves off, and get back on track.

EXTERMINATE THE ANTS

In the early stages especially, your own mind can be your worst enemy, constantly slipping ANTs (Automatic Negative Thoughts) in your jogging pants and telling you "you can't do it," "you'll never succeed," or just "don't bother." To combat negativity, write down your goals and regularly refer back to them. List the benefits of good health and stick them on the fridge door among your inspirational fridge magnets. Most important, plan to succeed by making your goals realistic and incremental. Perhaps draw up a mind map with your main goal as the central circle linked to the various activities or stages that are going to help you achieve your ultimate aim.

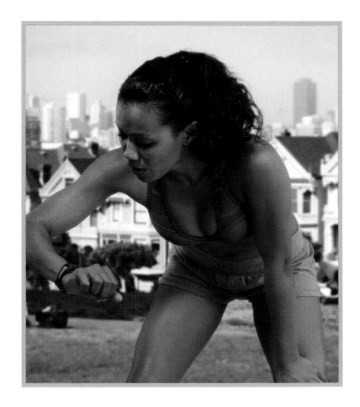

can check your resting heart rate right now. Just press your index and middle fingers onto the side of your neck in the soft, hollow area next to your windpipe. Once you can clearly feel your pulse, check your watch and count the beats for a period of six seconds. Whatever number you come up with (it will usually fall between 6 and 10) multiply it by 10. The final figure you come up with is, of course, the number of beats per minute (bpm). In the average adult, the resting heart rate will be between 60 and 100 bpm. Athletes may have a resting heart rate as low as 40 bpm. If your heart rate is continuously over 120 bpm or below 40 bpm, it is worth contacting your doctor to check whether or not this is normal for you.

THE ROLE OF THE HEART

The heart lies at the center of the cardiovascular system, so it is also central to life. Blood distributes nourishment from the digestive system and hormones from glands, constantly replenishing the body's supply of nutrients. Blood supplies oxygen from the lungs to the other organs and tissues and transports harmful carbon dioxide to the lungs, from where it is expelled into the air as we exhale. Similarly, our immune-system cells travel through the bloodstream, seeking out viruses and other harmful aliens. And, as if that weren't enough, the blood delivers your body's waste products to the kidneys and liver to be processed and unceremoniously ejected in urine and fecal matter.

CRUNCH SOME NUMBERS

Check your resting heart rate. This is a particularly useful number because it will increase considerably as you exercise and— perhaps most important—the speed at which your heartbeat returns to this resting state after activity is a very good indication of the state of your overall fitness. If you've been sitting reading this for at least five minutes, you

JOIN THE DIGITAL REVOLUTION

Or, you can save yourself the number crunching and invest in some digital technology that will do the job for you without the need to exercise your math skills. Wearable devices in the form of wristbands, watches and earphones are designed to automatically track such things as your physical activity, mood, and sleep patterns. These devices can be expensive, but they're getting cheaper ,and they're actually pretty good value when you consider how they can help to motivate you towards a healthier lifestyle. If money is tight, there is also a plethora of free apps designed to help with specific health goals, such as to quit smoking, reduce excessive drinking, lose weight, and eat healthily. The hugely popular 7 Minute Workout app is an international hit that has millions of people kick-starting their metabolism with a series of 12 specially selected exercises that can be completed with no equipment other than a sturdy chair or bench suitable for Step-Ups and Triceps Dips.

Many devices not only track your heart rate, but also track calories burned and signal you when you are at maximum exertion levels or have hit your optimal fat-burning zone.

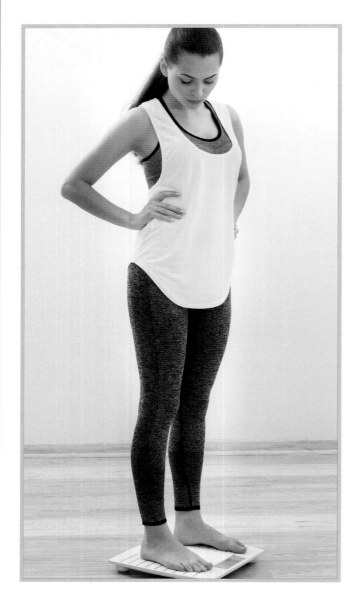

- *ENDURANCE* (60 to 70 percent) In this zone, your body burns stored fat as fuel. This might be your target zone if your goals are endurance and weight loss.
- *AEROBIC* (70 to 80 percent) In this zone, your body burns mostly fat and carbs. This might be your target zone if your goals are overall cardio fitness, weight management, and increased muscle strength.
- *ANEROBIC* (80 to 90 percent) In this zone, you will breathe heavily and feel your muscles tire. This might be your target zone if your goals are to increase lung capacity and lactate tolerance.

CHECK ALL YOUR VITALS
Keeping your blood pressure, blood sugar, cholesterol, and triglycerides in check is also important for heart health. Visit your doctor for a simple blood test and health check to find your current levels, and set your sights on matching the optimal levels for your gender and age group.

SET REALISTIC GOALS
Once you have the numbers you need and your long-term optimal targets are set you can get to work in earnest. If you're a young athlete, you can jump right in and start selecting the exercises you want to do today from the main sections in the book, adding them to your repertoire of healthy activities. If you're reading this because your doctor has informed you that you are clinically obese (see box on BMI) or your cholesterol level or blood pressure is too high, then you have to plan accordingly and begin by attempting one or two of the easiest exercises. The good news, or rather the terrible news, is that you are not alone, obesity has reached epidemic proportions in the United States and two thirds of American adults are either overweight or obese. Since the early 1990s the proportion of Americans who are clinically obese has soared by 75 percent. Heart disease, too, has risen steadily in recent times, especially in industrialized countries, due largely to changes

CALCULATE YOUR TARGET ZONE
It is essential to determine the optimal heart rate target zone for your specific fitness goal. The first step to figuring this out is to calculate your maximum heart rate (MHR). A rough, simple method is to subtract your age from the number 220 (MHR = 220 – your age). More precise formulas are based on gender and age: 216 – 93 percent of your age for men and 200 – 67 percent of your age for women.

There are four heart rate zones: endurance, aerobic, anaerobic, and VO_2 max. VO_2 max is the highest zone, but it is really just for elite athletes who can perform at nearly 100 percent for short, intense bursts of activity.

CALCULATING BMI

Body mass index (BMI)* is a measure of body fat based on height and weight that applies to adult men and women. You can use this chart to estimate your BMI. A high BMI can be an indicator of high body fatness.

WEIGHT	100	105	110	115	120	125	130	135	140	145	150	155	160	165	170	175	180	185	190	195	200	205	210	215
HEIGHT		Underweight					Healthy					Overweight					Obese				Extremely Obese			
5'0"	19	20	21	22	23	24	25	26	27	28	29	30	31	32	33	34	35	36	37	38	39	40	41	42
5'1"	18	19	20	21	22	23	24	25	26	27	28	29	30	31	32	33	34	35	36	36	37	38	39	40
5'2"	18	19	20	21	22	22	23	24	25	26	27	28	29	30	31	32	32	32	33	34	35	36	37	38
5'3"	17	18	19	20	21	22	23	24	24	25	25	26	27	28	29	30	31	32	32	33	34	35	36	37
5'4"	17	18	19	20	21	22	23	24	24	25	26	27	28	29	30	31	32	32	33	34	35	36	37	38
5'5"	16	17	18	19	20	20	21	22	23	24	25	25	26	27	28	29	30	30	31	32	33	34	35	35
5'6"	16	17	17	18	19	20	21	21	22	23	24	25	25	26	27	28	29	29	30	31	32	33	34	34
5'7"	15	16	17	18	18	19	20	21	22	22	23	24	25	25	26	27	28	29	29	30	31	31	33	33
5'8"	15	16	16	17	18	19	19	20	21	22	22	23	24	25	25	26	27	28	28	29	30	31	32	32
5'9"	14	15	16	17	17	18	19	20	20	21	22	22	23	24	25	25	26	27	28	28	29	30	31	31
5'10"	14	15	15	16	17	18	18	19	20	20	21	22	23	23	24	25	25	26	27	28	28	29	30	30
5'11"	14	14	15	16	16	17	18	18	19	20	21	21	22	23	23	24	25	25	26	27	28	28	29	30
6'0"	13	14	14	15	16	17	17	18	19	19	20	21	21	22	23	23	24	25	25	26	27	27	28	29
6'1"	13	13	14	15	15	16	17	17	18	19	19	20	21	21	22	23	23	24	25	25	26	27	27	28

According to the Centers for Disease Control and Prevention, BMI can be used to screen for weight categories that may lead to health problems but it is not diagnostic of the body fatness or health of an individual.

in diet and more sedentary lifestyles. Heart disease is now the leading cause of death for both men and women in the United States, claiming almost 700,000 lives every year.

SHED THOSE EXTRA POUNDS, DITCH THAT GUT
Even if you're not obese, but are still overweight, it can adversely effect your health and sense of well- being. And you don't need to check your BMI or anything else to know whether your happy or not when you see your reflection in a mirror or a shop window. Losing weight can improve your mental health and make you feel more confident. Excess belly fat particularly has been linked to higher blood pressure and unhealthy blood lipid levels. If you're burdened by a classic "spare tiyre" or "beer belly," it's time to shed some weight. Losing weight is not rocket science, it's just a matter of consuming fewer calories than you burn. Of course, it does require willpower for those of us who are fond of desserts. And, of course, the quality of the food is just as important as the quality. This is what we'll look at in more detail in the next couple of pages.

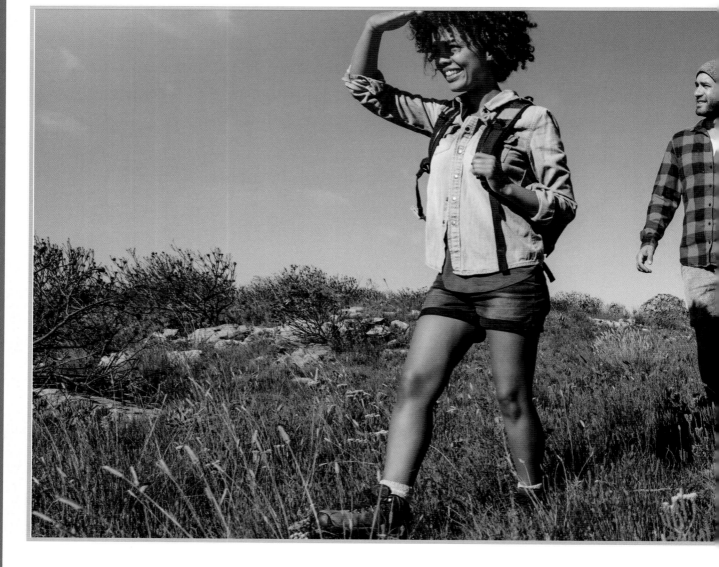

GET ACTIVE, GET FIT

To get healthy and remain that way, adults aged 18 to 64 should be performing at least two and a half hours of moderate aerobic exercise each week. If 150 minutes of physical activity a week seems daunting, don't despair. Once again, set yourself realistic targets that you know you can achieve and build up to the recommended amount over time. And perhaps it won't seem so bad when you consider that you can break it down into 10-minute sessions throughout the day and build up from there.

It will also help to consider that moderate aerobic activity is actually a walk in the park, quite literally, and, okay, maybe walking a little more briskly than you're used to. Fitness shouldn't be boring. Focus on activities you genuinely enjoy. Let your inner child loose by enjoying an evening of basketball or laser tag. Dust off your rollerblades (and protective gear), or join a tennis club and play doubles if that's your thing. If you're a keen gardener then you'll be pleased to know that pushing a lawn mower also counts (that's pushing, not driving!).

On top of the aerobic stuff, the fun stuff, you also need to perform anaerobic (strength) exercises on at least two days a week. The strength exercises need to work all the major muscle groups: shoulders, chest, back, abdomen, hips, legs, and arms.

Exercise is essential for good heart health, and once you start to enjoy good healthy exercise, you'll find yourself sneaking it in at every opportunity. You'll take the stairs instead of the

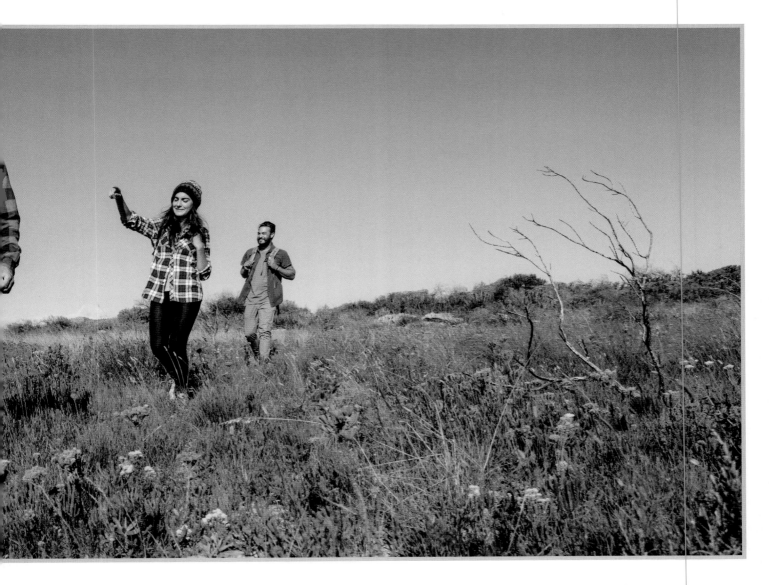

elevator. You'll find yourself playing with your kids in the park, instead of just watching them. You'll find yourself enjoying a romantic walk along the beach with your partner. You're on a virtuous cycle leading to ever improving health and fitness.

NO BUTTS ABOUT IT: STOP SMOKING

There are many steps you can take to help protect the health of your heart and arteries but avoiding tobacco is one of the best, which is why it's right here up front. Smoking is "the leading cause of preventable death and disease in the United States," according to the Centers for Disease Control and Prevention (CDC). Smokers are up to six times more likely to suffer a heart attack than nonsmokers, and the risk increases with the number of cigarettes smoked on a

daily basis. Not surprisingly, if you smoke or use other tobacco products, all reputable health organizations, including the American Heart Association (AHA) strongly advise you to quit. Quitting smoking can make a huge difference not only to your heart and lungs, but also to your overall health and happiness.

If you regularly smoke cannabis with tobacco in those states where the drug is legal, you're likely to get addicted to nicotine and may develop tobacco-related illnesses, such as cancer and coronary heart disease. If you use cannabis regularly it all too frequently makes you demotivated, paranoid, and uninterested in other things going on in your life, such as education, work, or fitness. The withdrawal symptoms you will experience when giving up nicotine or cannabis are more than

EAT WELL, STAY WELL

So, your heart is the body's engine room, pumping the blood that transports essential nutrients. But what exactly are those nutrients? And why are they "essential." Essential nutrients are simply those that cannot be supplied by the cells in our bodies and which must therefore be supplied by the food we consume. They are the proteins, vitamins, and minerals we need to maintain good health and the carbs and fats that supply energy.

Good nutrition, along with physical activity and relaxation, is a key factor in preventive health care. Basically, if you want your heart to be healthy and you want help it keep the rest of your body in good shape, you have to give it the right tools to work with. Legendary fitness guru Jack LaLanne, who died in 2011 aged 96, famously said: "Exercise is king and nutrition is queen" and a happy marriage between the two is all important for good health. In the 1950s, Jack was among the first to set America on track toward good health with his motivational talks and long-running TV show. And he walked the walk: with seemingly boundless energy he regularly performed feats of almost superhuman strength. Justly hailed as "the Godfather of Fitness," he

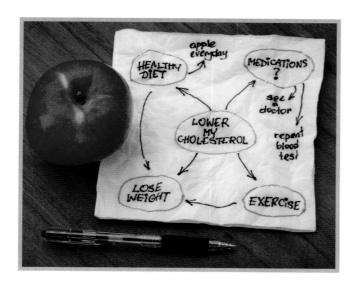

kept his optimism, energy, and razor-sharp wit until the very end of his long and productive life. Unlike Jack, we can't all begin the day with a two-hour workout, but we can all take his advice on healthy eating and make time for a hearty breakfast and a wholesome lunch and dinner.

BALANCING ACT

There is overwhelming scientific evidence showing that increasing our intake of certain nutrients not only increases our chances of enjoying optimum health, but also helps prevent certain diseases. For example, a group of vitamins and minerals known as antioxidants are believed to play a vital role in protecting our bodies against coronary heart disease, as well as some forms of cancer and other degenerative diseases. I think we all know by now that good eating is about "balance." But what should be balanced with what? And why does the advice change so frequently?

Well the good news is that there isn't space here to go into all the details of each specific nutrient, and the really good news is that you really don't need to know the details. The key thing to remember is to enjoy lots of variety in your diet with a selection of foods from the major groups as shown in the food pyramid (see left): cereals and potatoes, fruit and vegetables, protein foods, dairy products, and minimal sugars and fats. The words "enjoy" and "variety"

THE FOOD PYRAMID

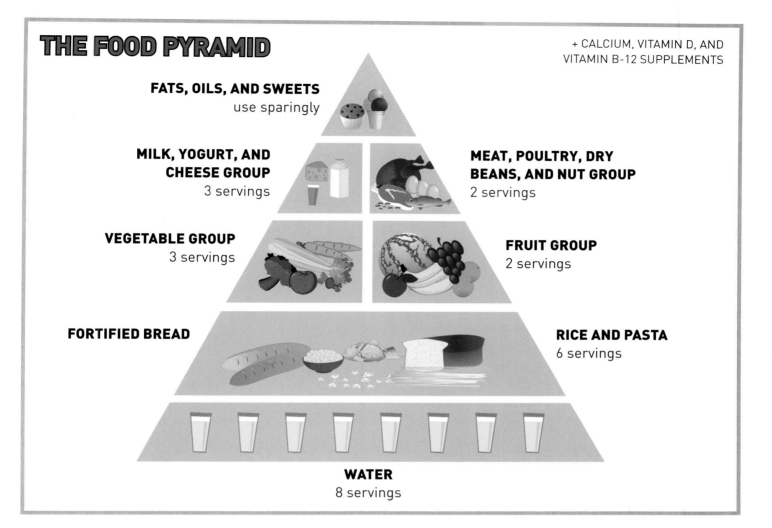

+ CALCIUM, VITAMIN D, AND VITAMIN B-12 SUPPLEMENTS

FATS, OILS, AND SWEETS
use sparingly

MILK, YOGURT, AND CHEESE GROUP
3 servings

MEAT, POULTRY, DRY BEANS, AND NUT GROUP
2 servings

VEGETABLE GROUP
3 servings

FRUIT GROUP
2 servings

FORTIFIED BREAD

RICE AND PASTA
6 servings

WATER
8 servings

are equally important here. Once you start to explore flavors and appreciate the wholesome tastes of the pyramid's "foundation foods," a whole world of culinary delight awaits you.

Top 10 Tips for Striking a Balance
- Eat a variety of foods.
- Cut down on sugar.
- Cut down on salt.
- Avoid eating too much fat.
- Avoid overcooking food to preserve vitamin and mineral content.
- Keep alcohol intake to sensible limits.
- Enjoy home cooking with fresh ingredients.
- Eat the right amount for you (to maintain a healthy body weight).
- Enjoy plenty of starch and fiber.
- Drink two liters of water each day.

SWEET TEMPTATION

Sure, Jack LaLanne once joked that if something tastes good you should "spit it out," but he was most referring to our nation's unhealthy addiction to sugar and saturated fat—the evil twins of the nutrient world. The popular press seems to change its mind constantly about which of the two is Public Health Enemy Number One when it comes to food products. The fact is, in excess, both are seriously detrimental to your health. You don't need to add any sugar to your diet; and if you eat a lot of processed food, you are almost certainly already getting a lot more sugar than you need. For example, when manufacturers boast of their "reduced fat" product, a peek at the ingredients often reveals that sugar has been added to compensate. Also, bear in mind that reducing quantities from sky high to high, doesn't help much. Get in the habit of checking ingredients on food labels before buying processed goods.

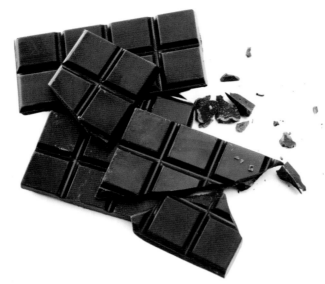

CHOCOLATE'S DARK SECRET

For chocoholics out there it's not all bad news: dark chocolate not only tastes delicious, it contains flavonoids that are actually beneficial for your heart. These compounds are believed to help reduce inflammation and lower your risk of heart disease. So if you really need to indulge your sweet tooth occasionally, sink it

SAY NO TO SALT

When it comes to heart health, it turns out that the evil twins—Sugar and Fat—have a big brother: Salt. Sure, we need salt to maintain good health: six grams or one teaspoonful per day for the average adult. Consuming too much salt, however, dramatically increases the risk of high blood pressure, which is a major health threat that can lead to a stroke or heart attack. And, remember, the six-gram daily quota doesn't mean you can sprinkle a teaspoonful of salt over your dinner (which, by the way, too many of us do!), that figure includes the salt that occurs naturally in many foods at trace levels and, crucially, that which is added in abundance to many processed foods. Once again, it's worth checking labels to see how much salt each food product contains. This may be labeled as a percentage of your daily requirement or in grams—you might be surprised by what you discover concerning the level of salt in some of your favorite foods. And don't forget that salt is often labeled by it's chemical name: sodium or sodium chloride.

VITAMINS: TOO MUCH OF A GOOD THING?

With the exception of vitamin D, which is produced by exposing the skin to sunlight, vitamins cannot be made by the body and have to be provided by food. Although it is highly unlikely that the amount of nutrients absorbed from food could reach dangerous levels, it can be detrimental to your health to fortify your diet with excessive amounts of certain supplements, such as vitamins A and D. Your doctor may advise you to take supplements under special circumstance (during pregnancy, for example), but otherwise don't buy them. For your heart, vitamin E is especially important in the fight to prevent heart disease. Once again, however, it is best to ingest it naturally through

GET FRESH!

Where possible, eat fresh food rather than processed foods with their added salt, sugar, and other chemical preservatives, colorings, and flavorings. Fresh fruit, vegetables, and salads are the superfoods of nutrition. Along with grain foods and potatoes, they should form the largest part of your diet, and the famed five-a-day rule should be seen as an absolute minimum. Apart from the benefits to your heart and the protection against damaging free radicals, the fiber in fruit and vegetables helps the bowel work more efficiently, and the vitamin C helps the body absorb iron. Make sure that you include leafy greens, too. Popeye was right, superfoods such as spinach and kale provide an abundance of beta-carotene, vitamin C, and folic acid (which is vital for the formation of new cells and is particularly important for pregnant women). And we can't mention Popeye without giving olive oil a mention too—an excellent source of heart-helping vitamin E. And, remember, healthy eating isn't just about finding the right kind of food; the way you prepare your food affects its nutritional value and calorie count. A portion of boiled potatoes, for example, contains around 100 calories of healthy carbs; but if you roast the same quantity, you'll end up with double the calories!

KEEP YOUR PROTEINS LEAN

Meat and poultry play a very important role in our diets and can be excellent sources of proteins, iron, and zinc. But keep a careful eye on your fat intake as animal foods tend to be high in saturated fat. Choose lean cuts where possible and trim away excess fat as required. Game meats such as venison and rabbit are lower in fat. Free-range chicken breast is a more wholesome option to enjoy with salad for a healthy lunch.

Your best bet for a healthy heart, however, is to limit your consumption of red meat and replace it with fish. Eating a diet rich in omega-3 fatty acids can also help ward off heart disease and many fish, including salmon, tuna, sardines, and herring, are great sources of omega-3. Aim to eat responsibly-sourced fish at least twice a week. Finally, nuts and seeds should be included in a varied diet—especially if you don't eat meat. Almonds, walnuts, and sunflower seeds, for example, are packed with protein, complex carbohydrates, iron, calcium, zinc, selenium, and vitamin E. Including them in your diet can help lower your risk of cardiovascular disease, but be sure to keep serving sizes small because they're also packed with calories.

PLAN YOUR MEALS

To put all this into practice, you need to plan your meals carefully. Your meal plan forms the basis of your weekly shopping list so that you buy all the right ingredients and avoid having stuff rotting in the bottom of your fridge—it's estimated that one in every five bags of shopping in the United States ends up in the garbage! You're also less likely to be suckered by eye-catching packaging into buying stuff you don't need and which isn't good for you.

DON'T SKIP BREAKFAST

Jack LaLanne once asked, "Would you get your dog up in the morning for coffee and a donut?" Jack was referring to the increasing tendency for busy Americans to "grab a bite" for breakfast or skip it entirely, relying solely

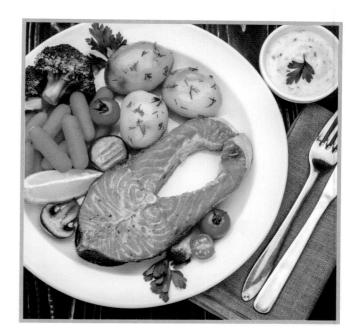

on coffee to kick-start the day. Jack lived by the old adage, "breakfast like a king, lunch like a prince, and dine like a pauper." He was a great believer in the benefits of juicing for aiding digestion and packing nutrients into a single morning drink. For a heart-healthy breakfast, reach for whole grains, such as oatmeal, whole-grain cereals, or whole-wheat toast. Choose good sources of protein, such as eggs, salmon, or a small serving of nuts or peanut butter. Include calcium-rich dairy products, such as milk, yogurt, or cheese. And get a helping of fruit and vegetables, which can be enjoyed as a smoothie. By contrast, the final meal of the day should be relatively light so that your digestive system doesn't have to go into overdrive while you sleep. A typical evening meal for Jack would be a salad with fresh fish and brown rice. But meal times aren't just about stocking up on nutrients; meal times should be a pleasure and an opportunity to relax and catch up with family and friends. The importance of relaxation in maintaining a healthy heart should not be underestimated.

TOP UP WITH WATER

Make sure you drink plenty of water throughout the day. Apart from keeping you hydrated, it helps keep your skin clear and curbs hunger pangs so you don't feel the need to snack between meals.

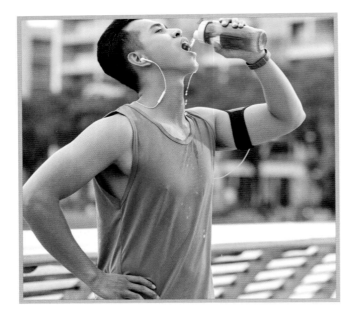

If you find plain water too bland, squeeze in a bit of lemon juice. Watermelons, peaches, and cucumbers are also excellent sources of H2O. Keep a liter bottle of water on your desk as a reminder to take water on board throughout the day. The average adult should be drinking two liters a day.

RAISE A GLASS

According to some scientific studies, moderate consumption of alcohol can actually help raise your levels of HDL, or good cholesterol. It can also help prevent blood-clot formation and artery damage. Red wine in particular may offer benefits for your heart. Excessive alcohol intake, however, increases your risk of a fatal stroke or heart attack. As with all things, the key is moderation. Good health!

KEEP YOUR LIFE IN BALANCE

Over the years a vast body of scientific evidence has emerged to verify what we instinctively already know: stress, anxiety, and anger all impact negatively on our health as well as our mood. Continuous stress can ultimately lead to high blood pressure and an increased risk of heart disease and stroke. The flipside of this coin is a lot brighter—maintaining a positive outlook on life and learning to relax can help you stay happier and healthier for longer.

Heavy workloads and a cantankerous boss, a long commute in heavy traffic, the struggle to make ends meet, and the endless bombardment of advertisements telling you that you need this or that to make your life easier—who has time to exercise and eat well? Once again, the answer is that you make time. Plan for a healthier work/life balance and stay positive by taking positive steps, however small, to get a little more organized and to gradually replace bad habits with good ones. Smoking half a pack of cigarettes and then throwing the other half a way in disgust and self-loathing, only to buy another pack the next day, is dumb right? And expensive! It's the positive steps that actually work and make you feel good about yourself: actively seeking support from your local stop-smoking service, starting nicotine replacement therapy, going out for a brisk walk when you feel the need for a cigarette instead of giving in to the nicotine-induced craving. The same approach applies to all aspects of your life: stay positive and take positive action!

COUNT TO TEN

"Damn braces, bless relaxes," chirped the British artist and poet William Blake. In modern terminology, that means that when you drive, for instance, instead of exchanging curses with that idiot who just cut you off in rush-hour traffic, breathe deeply, and count to ten. You may not be able to take Blake's advice literally and give your blessing to everyone and every thing that irritates you, but it might help to know that you're only doing yourself harm if you allow yourself to become angry. People who respond to negative situations with anger are three times more likely to suffer from heart disease and five times more likely to have a heart attack before turning 55. Use the time in your car positively by listening to relaxing music or a podcast of your favorite comedy program and you'll be less likely to fire up when you see someone driving badly. Before you know it, you'll be looking forward to your drive to work for the opportunity of a little "me time," and you may find yourself skipping the highway and taking the longer scenic route to gain maximum benefit from your newfound four-fendered friend.

"WHEN HEARTS ARE HIGH, THE TIME WILL FLY"
The same positivity can be applied to other things in life that you deem to be obligations, and which you aren't supposed to enjoy. Doing the housework, for example, may not be as invigorating as a step class, but household chores do get you moving and can be a great opportunity to give your heart a little workout, while burning calories and actually lifting your spirits. Put your favorite music on and shimmy your way across the room as you dust and vacuum. We don't sing while washing the dishes any more—the electric dishwasher put paid to that—but your morning shower needn't be the last bastion of home operatics, you can still sing as you load the dishwasher and wipe down the work surfaces.

By the way, whether listening to a funny radio program or cracking jokes with your friends, laughter really is good medicine. According to the American Heart Association, laughter lowers stress hormones, which can decrease inflammation in your arteries and raise your levels of "good cholesterol."

And if you don't feel ready for a hearty belly laugh, you will be encouraged to learn that researchers have found that smiling, even it starts as a fake smile, can enhance positivity and actually benefit heart health. Smiling, like laughter, is highly contagious and if it takes a forced smile to get the ball rolling, so be it. A study from Penn State University found that people who smile appear to be more likeable, courteous, and competent, so a happy countenance will often bring better results at work as well as at play. Best of all, smiling is easy, its free, and it helps to lift that heavy weight from your shoulders. So it may well be that of all the muscles you work out today, the face muscles might just be the most important. That, in itself, is something to smile about.

GO OUT AND PLAY
Your work life needs to be balanced by play. So take your play time as seriously as you take your work. Find like-minded people by joining a club or a social group; the Internet has made this easier than ever before with online groups for every conceivable pastime, whether it's chess or the Charleston that floats your boat. Make time to learn to crochet or play the clarinet, build a doll's house or build a summer house, make model airplanes or learn to fly a real airplane. Okay, all of these options won't be realistic for everyone, but there is something for everyone and if you really don't know what that something is, have fun trying new things until you find out. Like Tom Waites says, "Fishing for a good time, starts with throwing in a line." Go fish.

REACH FOR GOOD HEART HEALTH
Yoga improves your balance, flexibility, and strength. Better still, it helps you relax and relieves stress, so reducing your risk of cardiovascular disease. This book contains many stretching exercises that will bring you the same benefits, but joining a yoga class is a great way to enhance your heart fitness and meet new friends.

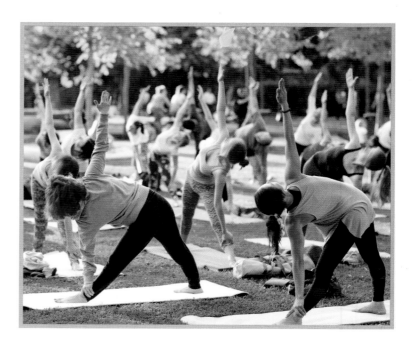

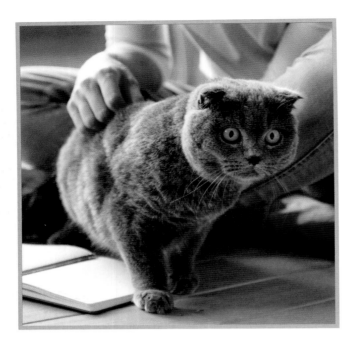

A STROKE THAT HELPS YOUR HEART?

As well as offering unconditional love, pets can come with major heart-health benefits and the National Institutes of Health (NIH) suggests that owning a pet may help lower your chances of dying from heart disease. Certainly, taking your dog for a daily walk boosts your fitness level, but it's interesting to note that even the simple act of stroking a cat is thought to be highly therapeutic, lowering your heart rate and stress levels.

TURN OFF, TUNE IN

For all the myriad benefits the internet and all our modern devices afford us, the endless noise from cyberspace, TV, and electronic advertising billboards can leave you feeling mentally saturated and stressed out. Escape to the countryside or the sea shore once in a while and "get away from it all." Turn off the screens, and tune in to the wonders of the natural world.

SLEEP ON IT!

And, remember, you have one great natural ally in the battle for optimum health and happiness—sleep! The average adult thrives on eight hours sleep. Forget those folk who insist that sleep is a waste of time and boast about getting by on, or even attributing their success to five hours or less. Napoleon is perhaps the most famous of these

doze dodgers and look what happened to him! Sleeping is not a waste of time. While you snooze, your body pushes on with healing any wear and tear, including essential maintenance work on your heart and blood vessels. Sleep affects how your body reacts to insulin, the hormone that controls your blood-sugar levels, which when too high can lead to diabetes. Sleep helps maintain a healthy immune system, which is why you're more likely to catch colds and other common infections when you've been burning the midnight oil.

It's not just your physical health that's enhanced; sleep also plays a vital role in your mental wellbeing. While you sleep, your brain is busy sorting out your memory bank, reinforcing important lessons learned during the day and clearing away mental clutter. Studies show that sleep enhances learning and performance, whether you're cramming for a science exam, cogitating about how best to close a business deal, learning to play a musical instrument, or just brushing up on your putting technique for golf. Sleep helps you to think clearly and stay focused. Bottom line: If Napoleon spent more time napping, he might not have woken up on that chilly morning and put "Invade Moscow" on his things-to-do-today list!

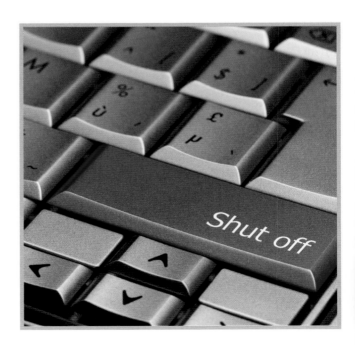

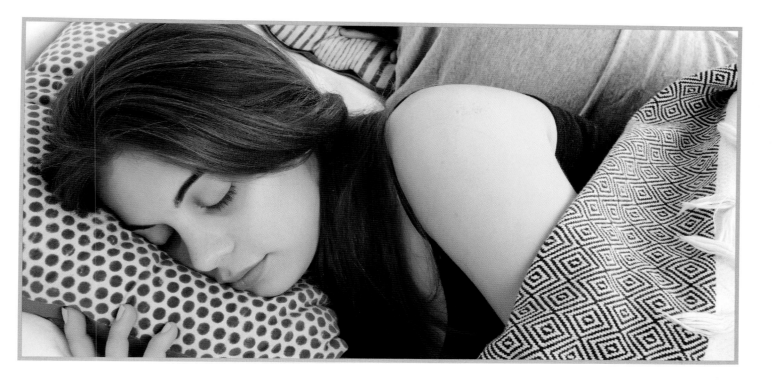

Top 10 Tips for a Good Night's Kip

Make sure that you do everything to promote a good night's sleep. Try these tips to make sure you get the refreshing sleep you need.

▸▸ *Have a sleep routine and stick to it.*
Staying up late and sleeping in will disrupt your body clock. Aim to limit alterations to your sleeping pattern to within an hour if you want to sleep in at weekends.

▸▸ *Be physically active during the day.*
As well as helping you to look and feel great during the day, a good workout will also help you sleep more soundly at night.

▸▸ *Create your dream bedroom.*
Keep your bedroom tidy and free from clutter and a sanctuary from all signs of daily strife. Banish computers or work-related items. Hang thick curtains and use low, dim lighting to keep your bedroom cool, dark, and sensual. The bedroom isn't just for sleeping, of course. A good workout between the sheets not only burns calories, it also relieves stress and promotes sleep.

▸▸ *Wind down before bedtime.*
Avoid computer and TV screens and use the last hour before sleep for quiet time. Listen to some music (Mozart not Motorhead) or make simple preparations for the next day. A relaxing hot bath is an ideal way to soak away your worries before slipping between the sheets.

▸▸ *Nap sparingly.*
Keep daytime naps to a maximum of 20 minutes. Although a brief siesta during the afternoon can reinvigorate your body, too much sleeping during the day will be counterproductive.

▸▸ *Avoid heavy meals too close to bedtime.*
If you feel hungry, have a banana and a glass of milk. Bananas are a good source of potassium and magnesium, which are natural muscle relaxants.

▸▸ *Avoid caffeine.*
Coffee and tea are best enjoyed in the morning and early afternoon. The stimulating effects of caffeine can last for up to eight hours, so your after-dinner coffee might prevent you from sleeping.

▸▸ *Don't drink too much too close to bedtime.*
To avoid the need for post-midnight trip to the bathroom, skip the late-night beverage. Keep a glass of water by your bed in case you wake up feeling thirsty.

▸▸ *Avoid bright lights.*
Read a chapter of a good novel, but avoid backlit devices: bright screens can actually overstimulate the mind and keep you awake for longer.

SECTION TWO

HEALTHY HEART WORKOUTS

Now that your understand the benefits of a healthy heart and have a wide range of options to try so that you can make your lifestyle even heart-health friendlier, it is time to get moving. In this section, you will find a series of Heart Healthy workouts divided by level of difficulty—representing beginner to advanced.

LEVEL ONE

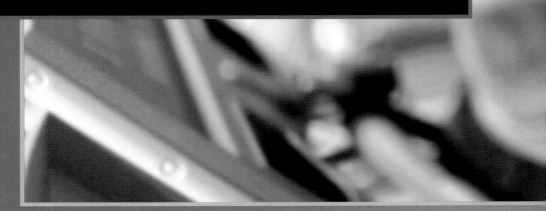

Start with the basics to introduce yourself to a heart-friendly workout program. Level One introduces you to this process, with three workouts that are suitable for beginners. You will work with your own body weight and with light resistance, such as hand weights, and you'll also be introduced to the Swiss ball, which adds a core-challenging element of instability to an exerice. You will also work with steps, which add an aerobic boost to your regimen.

As you master the exercises in this section and advance through the workouts, periodically check back to this page to see how are progressing toward the goals listed in the chart below. Once you have safely achieved all these milestones, you can move on to the workouts shown in Level Two.

LEVEL ONE PROGRESS REPORT

WORKOUT	NAME	GOAL
A	Intro to Strength Training	Increase full-body muscle strength
B	Cardio-Strength Combo	Improve full-body muscle strength and increase stamina and endurance
C	Full-Body Stretch Sequence	Improve flexibility and limberness

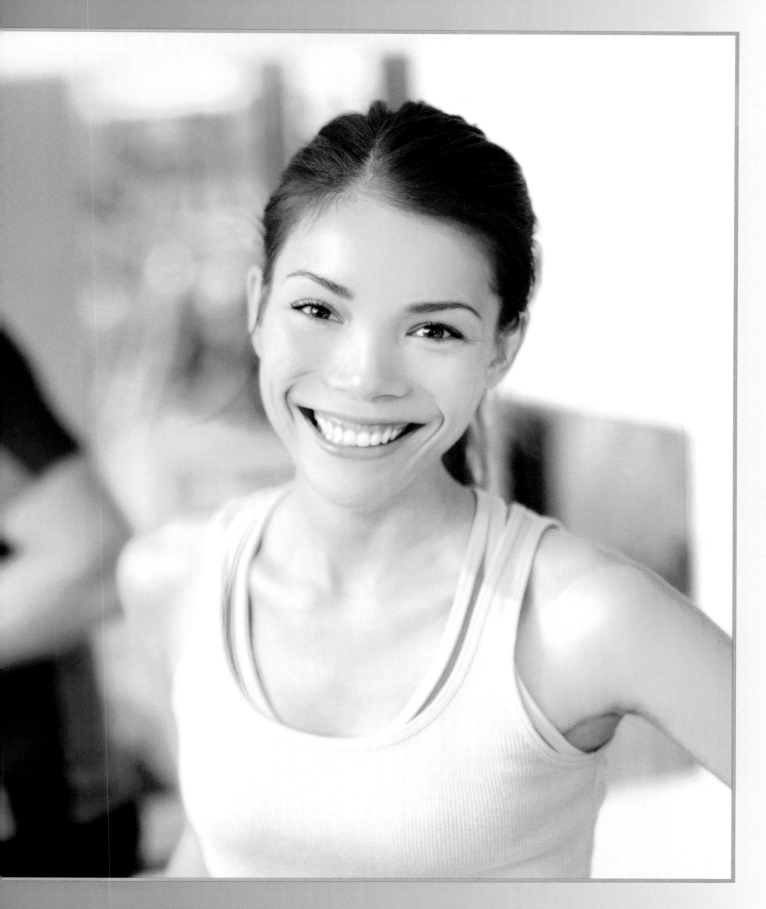

WORKOUT A

Intro to Strength Training

A healthy heart starts with a strong body, so it is necessary to include strength training in your Healthy Heat regimen. The Intro to Strength Training workout takes you through a series of exercises that call for you to use your own body weight as resistance and also introduces you to hand weights and the aerobic step. Concentrate on executing these exercises with good form as you learn to mindfully engage your muscles.

1. CHAIR SQUAT
(Pages 30–31)

Perform 10 repetitions.

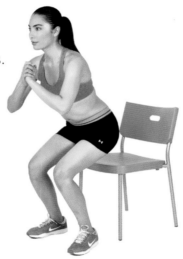

2. CHAIR PLIÉ
(Pages 32–33)

Perform 10 repetitions.

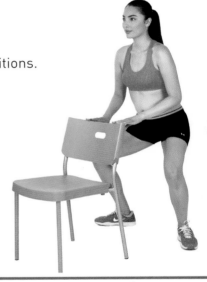

3. SINGLE-LEG BALANCE
(Pages 34–35)

Perform the entire sequence three times on each side.

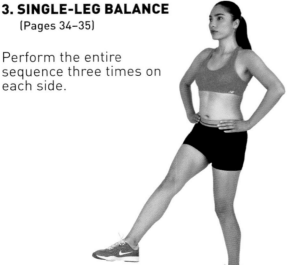

4. LATERAL STEP-AND-CURL
(Pages 36–37)

Perform two sets, alternating sides for 10 to 12 repetitions on each side.

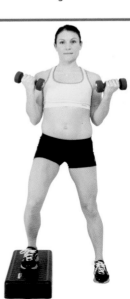

5. TINY STEP
Pages 38–39

Alternate legs for 10 repetitions on each side.

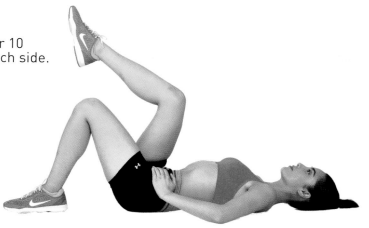

6. CHAIR POSE
(Pages 40–41)

Perform two repetitions, holding each for 30 seconds.

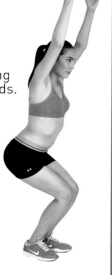

7. LATERAL LUNGE
(Pages 42–43)

Perform two sets of 10 repetitions on each side.

8. LATERAL-EXTENSION LATERAL LUNGE
(Pages 44–45)

Alternate sides for 10 to 12 repetitions on each side.

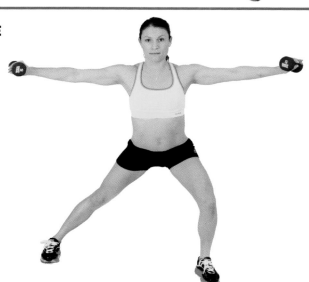

CHAIR SQUAT

1 Stand upright in front of the chair. Clasp your hands, and position them in front of your chest.

2 Slowly lower into a squat position.

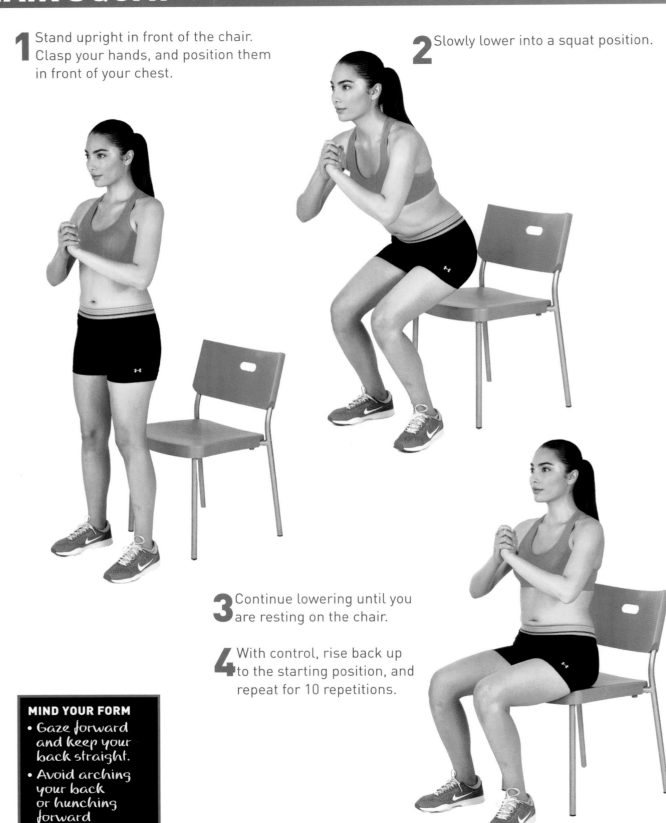

3 Continue lowering until you are resting on the chair.

4 With control, rise back up to the starting position, and repeat for 10 repetitions.

MIND YOUR FORM
- Gaze forward and keep your back straight.
- Avoid arching your back or hunching forward

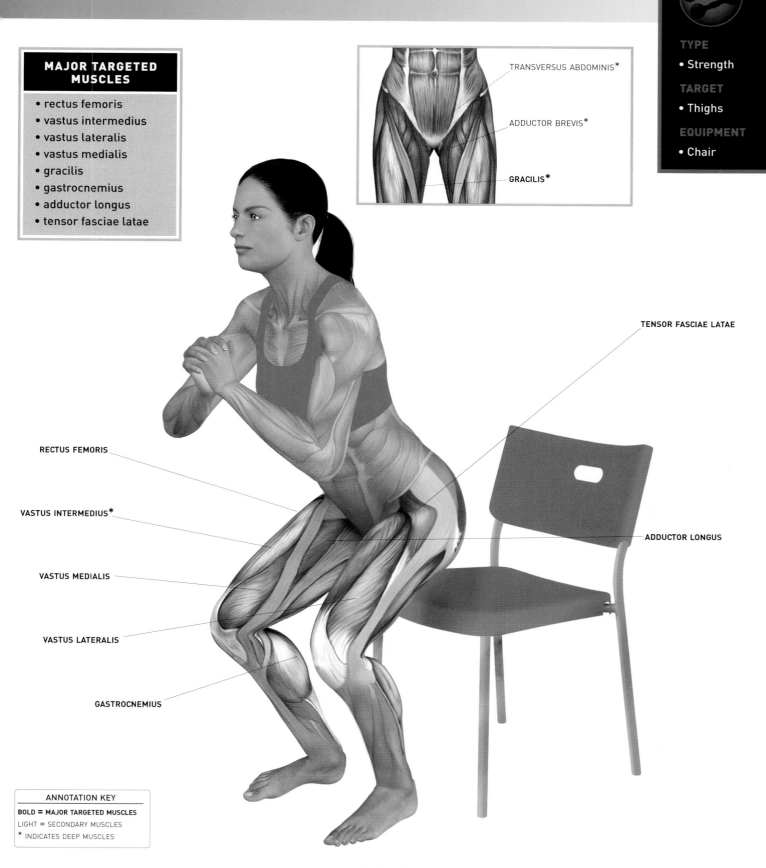

MAJOR TARGETED MUSCLES

- rectus femoris
- vastus intermedius
- vastus lateralis
- vastus medialis
- gracilis
- gastrocnemius
- adductor longus
- tensor fasciae latae

TRANSVERSUS ABDOMINIS*

ADDUCTOR BREVIS*

GRACILIS*

TYPE
- Strength

TARGET
- Thighs

EQUIPMENT
- Chair

TENSOR FASCIAE LATAE

RECTUS FEMORIS

VASTUS INTERMEDIUS*

ADDUCTOR LONGUS

VASTUS MEDIALIS

VASTUS LATERALIS

GASTROCNEMIUS

ANNOTATION KEY

BOLD = MAJOR TARGETED MUSCLES
LIGHT = SECONDARY MUSCLES
* INDICATES DEEP MUSCLES

CHAIR PLIÉ

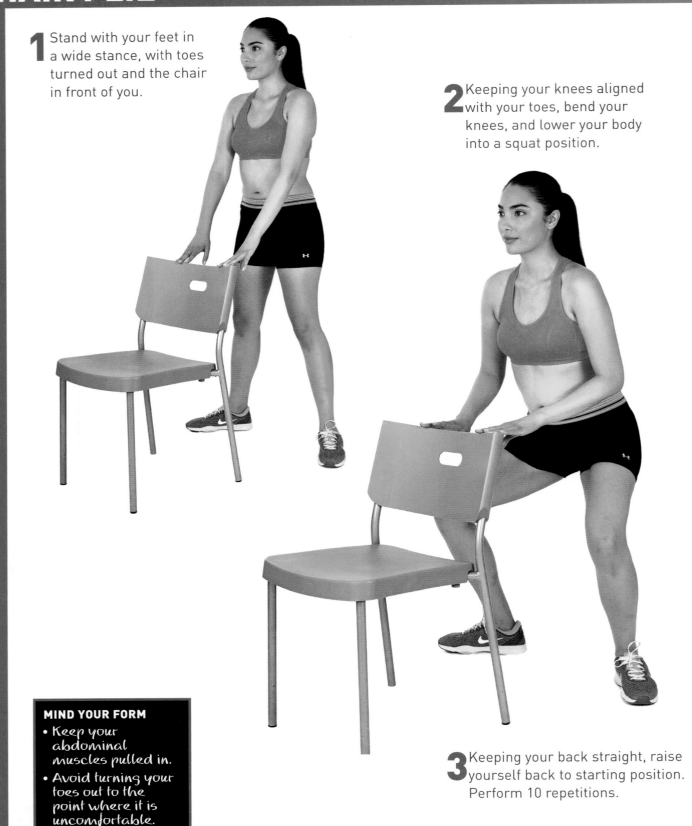

1 Stand with your feet in a wide stance, with toes turned out and the chair in front of you.

2 Keeping your knees aligned with your toes, bend your knees, and lower your body into a squat position.

3 Keeping your back straight, raise yourself back to starting position. Perform 10 repetitions.

MIND YOUR FORM
- Keep your abdominal muscles pulled in.
- Avoid turning your toes out to the point where it is uncomfortable.

TYPE
• Strength
TARGET
• Inner thighs
EQUIPMENT
• Chair

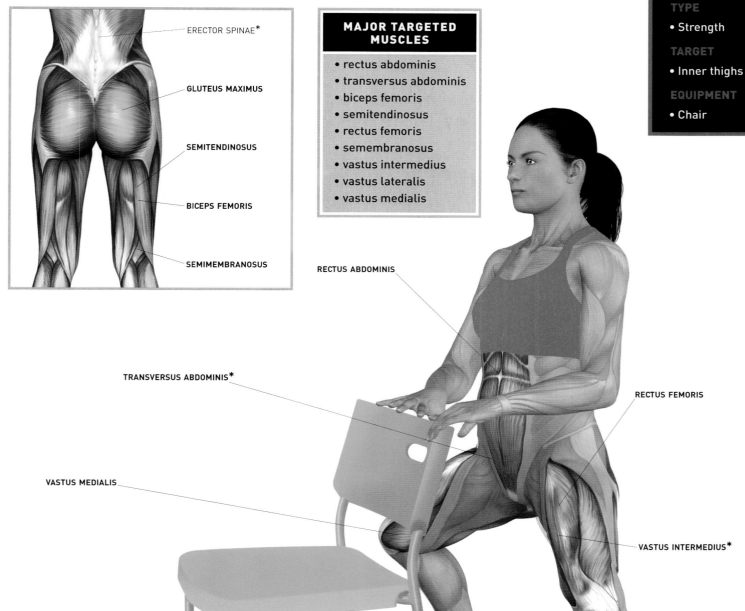

ERECTOR SPINAE*

GLUTEUS MAXIMUS

SEMITENDINOSUS

BICEPS FEMORIS

SEMIMEMBRANOSUS

MAJOR TARGETED MUSCLES

- rectus abdominis
- transversus abdominis
- biceps femoris
- semitendinosus
- rectus femoris
- semembranosus
- vastus intermedius
- vastus lateralis
- vastus medialis

RECTUS ABDOMINIS

TRANSVERSUS ABDOMINIS*

VASTUS MEDIALIS

RECTUS FEMORIS

VASTUS INTERMEDIUS*

VASTUS LATERALIS

ANNOTATION KEY
BOLD = MAJOR TARGETED MUSCLES
LIGHT = SECONDARY MUSCLES
* INDICATES DEEP MUSCLES

SINGLE-LEG BALANCE

1 Stand with your hands on your hips, and raise your right leg, bent at the knee, directly in front of you at a 90-degree angle. Hold for 15 seconds.

2 Press your right leg down and forward, though not touching the floor, and hold for 15 seconds.

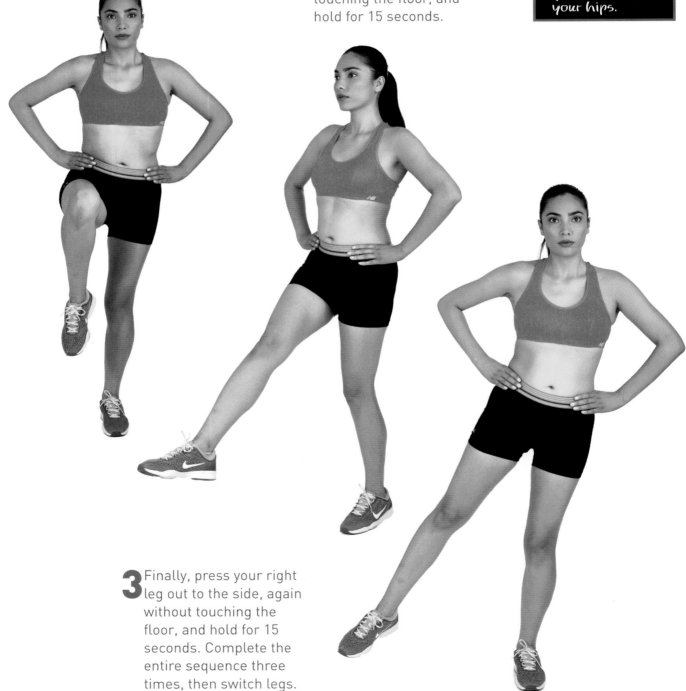

3 Finally, press your right leg out to the side, again without touching the floor, and hold for 15 seconds. Complete the entire sequence three times, then switch legs.

Section Two • Level One • Workout A

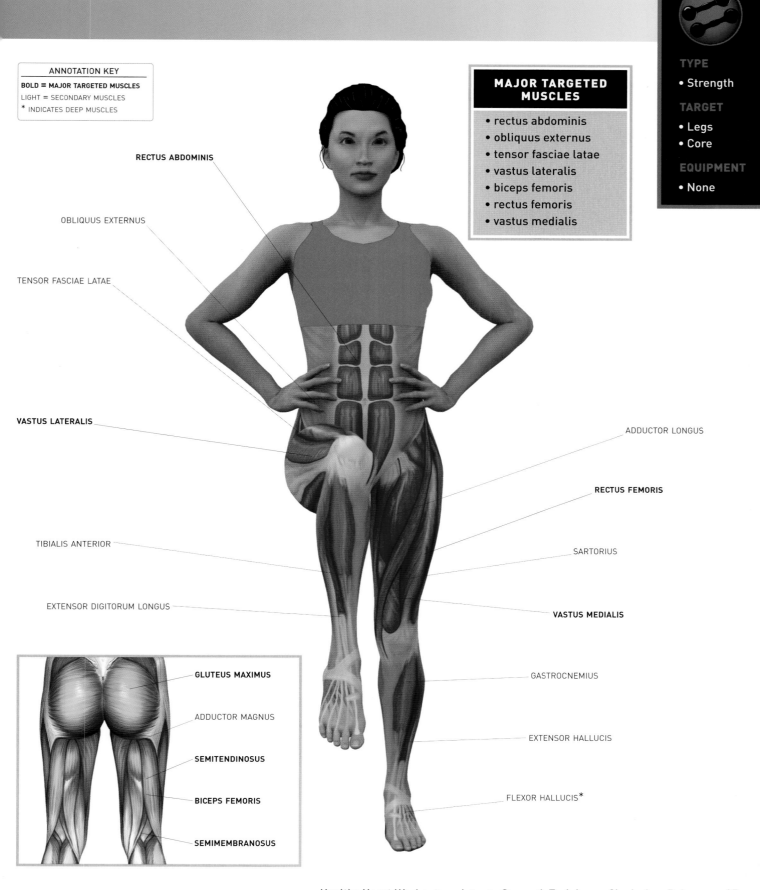

MAJOR TARGETED MUSCLES

- rectus abdominis
- obliquus externus
- tensor fasciae latae
- vastus lateralis
- biceps femoris
- rectus femoris
- vastus medialis

TYPE
- Strength

TARGET
- Legs
- Core

EQUIPMENT
- None

RECTUS ABDOMINIS

OBLIQUUS EXTERNUS

TENSOR FASCIAE LATAE

VASTUS LATERALIS

TIBIALIS ANTERIOR

EXTENSOR DIGITORUM LONGUS

ADDUCTOR LONGUS

RECTUS FEMORIS

SARTORIUS

VASTUS MEDIALIS

GASTROCNEMIUS

EXTENSOR HALLUCIS

FLEXOR HALLUCIS*

GLUTEUS MAXIMUS

ADDUCTOR MAGNUS

SEMITENDINOSUS

BICEPS FEMORIS

SEMIMEMBRANOSUS

LATERAL STEP-AND-CURL

1 Stand with your feet hip-width apart and your arms at your sides, a dumbbell in each hand and a step positioned beside your right foot.

2 Step to the right, placing your right foot on the step. Simultaneously bend your elbows, curling the dumbbells into your chest.

3 Lowering the dumbbells, bring your left leg onto the step so that your feet are together.

4 Curl the dumbbells into your chest as you step your right leg off the step. Release the dumbbells as you step down with your left leg. You should now be in the starting position with the step to your right.

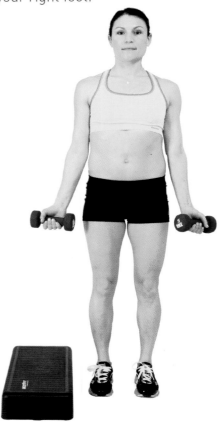

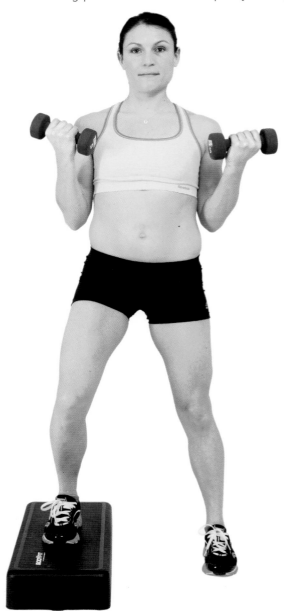

MIND YOUR FORM
- Keep your upper arms stationary as you curl and release.
- Keep your movements smooth and controlled.
- Keep your torso facing forward.
- Pull your abdominal muscles inward to keep them engaged.
- Gaze forward.
- Press your shoulders away from your ears.
- Avoid twisting your neck.
- Avoid hunching your shoulders.
- Avoid arching your back or hunching forward.
- Don't move so quickly that you sacrifice form.

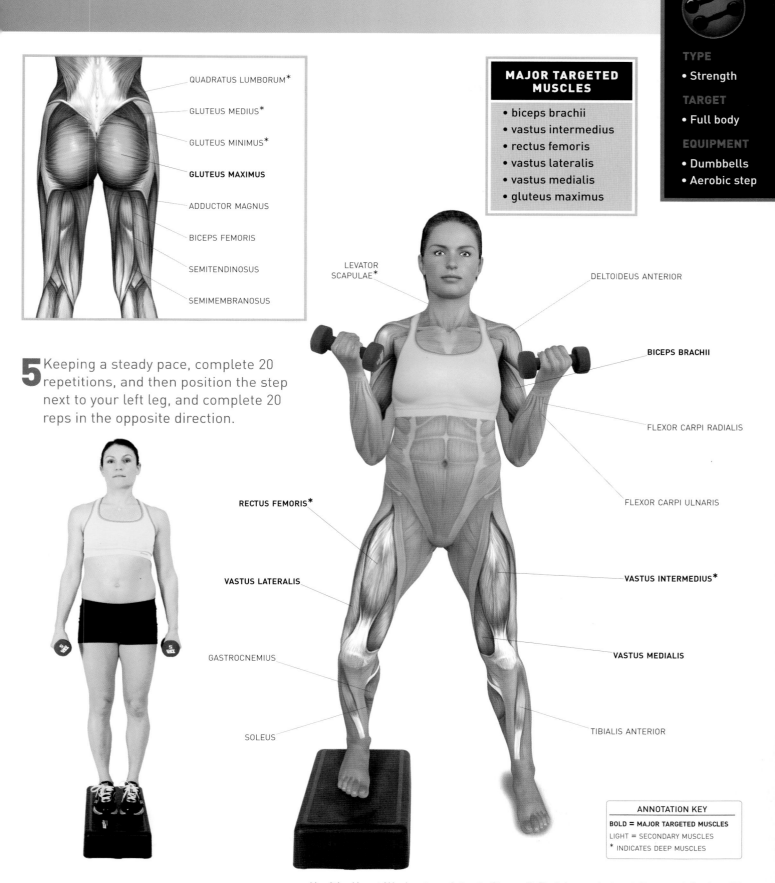

QUADRATUS LUMBORUM*

GLUTEUS MEDIUS*

GLUTEUS MINIMUS*

GLUTEUS MAXIMUS

ADDUCTOR MAGNUS

BICEPS FEMORIS

SEMITENDINOSUS

SEMIMEMBRANOSUS

MAJOR TARGETED MUSCLES

- biceps brachii
- vastus intermedius
- rectus femoris
- vastus lateralis
- vastus medialis
- gluteus maximus

TYPE
- Strength

TARGET
- Full body

EQUIPMENT
- Dumbbells
- Aerobic step

5 Keeping a steady pace, complete 20 repetitions, and then position the step next to your left leg, and complete 20 reps in the opposite direction.

LEVATOR SCAPULAE*

DELTOIDEUS ANTERIOR

BICEPS BRACHII

FLEXOR CARPI RADIALIS

FLEXOR CARPI ULNARIS

RECTUS FEMORIS*

VASTUS INTERMEDIUS*

VASTUS LATERALIS

VASTUS MEDIALIS

GASTROCNEMIUS

TIBIALIS ANTERIOR

SOLEUS

ANNOTATION KEY

BOLD = MAJOR TARGETED MUSCLES
LIGHT = SECONDARY MUSCLES
* INDICATES DEEP MUSCLES

TINY STEPS

1 Begin by lying on your back on a mat with your knees bent and your feet on tiptoes on the floor. Place your hands on your hipbones, and raise your left knee toward your chest while keeping your abdominals pulled in.

MIND YOUR FORM
- Keep your abdominals pulled in during the entire exercise.
- Correct action Increases lower-abdominal stability and helps protect the lower back.
- Avoid moving your hips throughout.

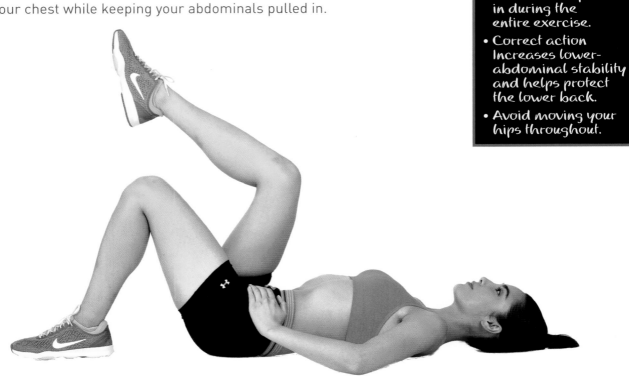

2 As you lower your left leg to the floor, keep your abdominals tightened, and hold for 10 seconds.

3 Switch legs, and repeat, alternating sides for 10 repetitions on each leg.

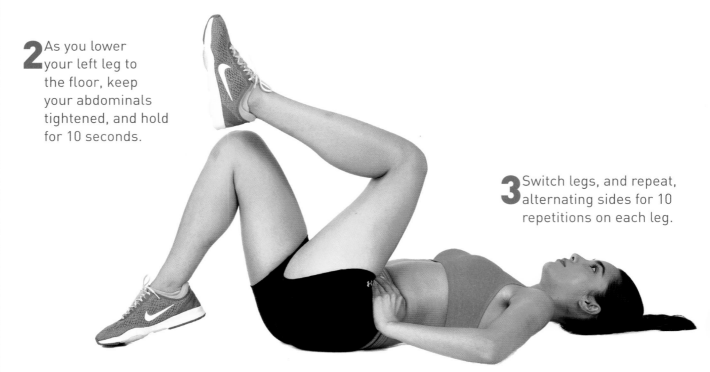

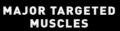

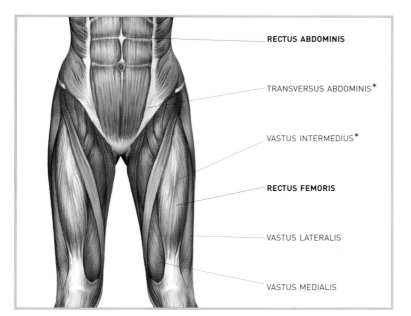

RECTUS ABDOMINIS

TRANSVERSUS ABDOMINIS*

VASTUS INTERMEDIUS*

RECTUS FEMORIS

VASTUS LATERALIS

VASTUS MEDIALIS

MAJOR TARGETED MUSCLES

• gluteus maximus
• tensor fasciae latae
• obliquus internus
• rectus femoris
• biceps femoris
• gluteus medius
• rectus abdominis

ANNOTATION KEY

BOLD = MAJOR TARGETED MUSCLES
LIGHT = SECONDARY MUSCLES
* INDICATES DEEP MUSCLES

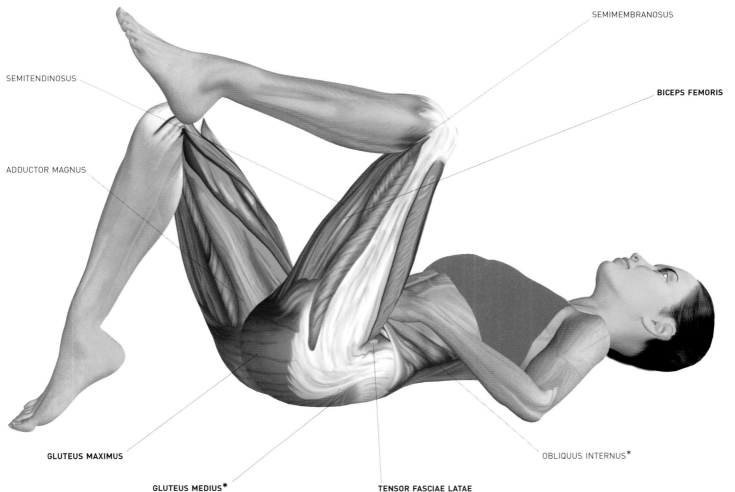

SEMIMEMBRANOSUS

SEMITENDINOSUS

BICEPS FEMORIS

ADDUCTOR MAGNUS

GLUTEUS MAXIMUS

OBLIQUUS INTERNUS*

GLUTEUS MEDIUS*

TENSOR FASCIAE LATAE

CHAIR POSE

1 Stand tall with your feet together and your arms at your sides.

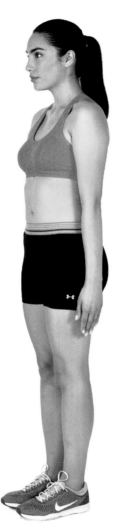

2 Bend your knees, and push your buttocks back while you simultaneously raise your arms over your head, being sure to maintain a flat back.

3 Keep your upper body one long length for 15 to 30 seconds. Release the pose, return to the starting position, and then repeat two times.

MIND YOUR FORM
• Avoid arching your back.
• Perform the lowering motion with only your thighs, knees, and hips to achieve the proper lower-body position.

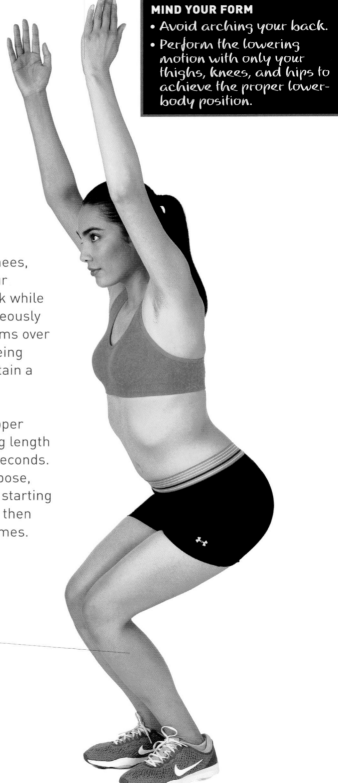

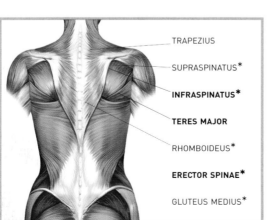

TRAPEZIUS

SUPRASPINATUS*

INFRASPINATUS*

TERES MAJOR

RHOMBOIDEUS*

ERECTOR SPINAE*

GLUTEUS MEDIUS*

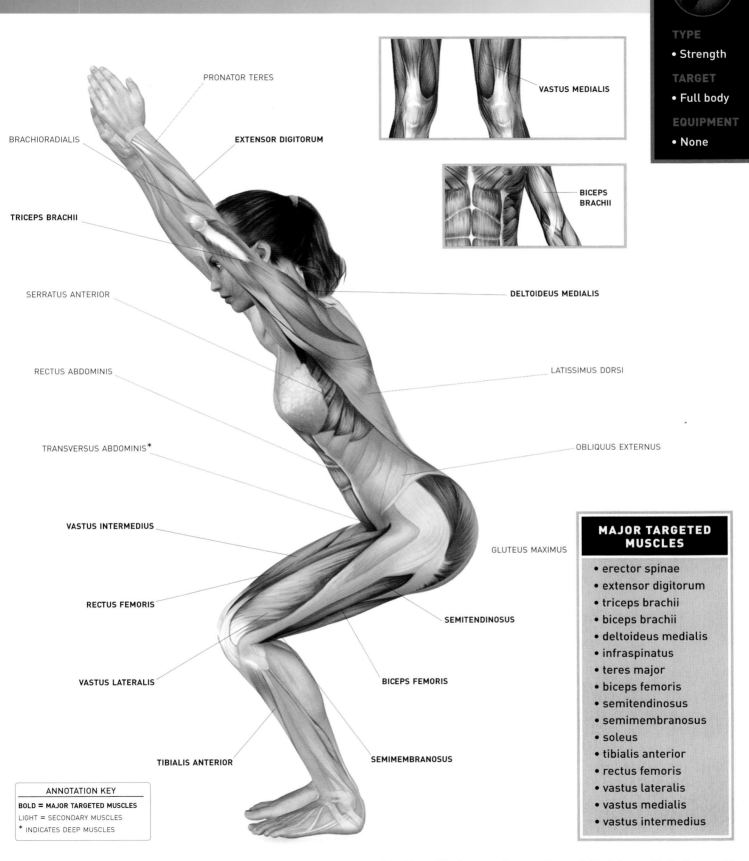

PRONATOR TERES

BRACHIORADIALIS

EXTENSOR DIGITORUM

TRICEPS BRACHII

SERRATUS ANTERIOR

RECTUS ABDOMINIS

TRANSVERSUS ABDOMINIS*

VASTUS INTERMEDIUS

RECTUS FEMORIS

VASTUS LATERALIS

TIBIALIS ANTERIOR

VASTUS MEDIALIS

BICEPS BRACHII

DELTOIDEUS MEDIALIS

LATISSIMUS DORSI

OBLIQUUS EXTERNUS

GLUTEUS MAXIMUS

SEMITENDINOSUS

BICEPS FEMORIS

SEMIMEMBRANOSUS

TYPE
• Strength
TARGET
• Full body
EQUIPMENT
• None

MAJOR TARGETED MUSCLES

- erector spinae
- extensor digitorum
- triceps brachii
- biceps brachii
- deltoideus medialis
- infraspinatus
- teres major
- biceps femoris
- semitendinosus
- semimembranosus
- soleus
- tibialis anterior
- rectus femoris
- vastus lateralis
- vastus medialis
- vastus intermedius

ANNOTATION KEY

BOLD = MAJOR TARGETED MUSCLES
LIGHT = SECONDARY MUSCLES
* INDICATES DEEP MUSCLES

LATERAL LUNGE

1 Stand with your feet wider than shoulder-width apart with your arms outstretched in front of you, parallel to the floor.

2 Step out to the left. Squat down on your right leg, bending at your hips, while maintaining a neutral spine. Begin to extend your left leg, keeping both feet flat on the floor.

3 Bend your right knee until your thigh is parallel to the floor and your left leg is fully extended.

4 Keeping your arms parallel to the floor, squeeze your glutes, and press off your right leg to return to the starting position, and

MIND YOUR FORM
- Keep your bent knee aligned with your toes.
- Keep your spine in a neutral position as you bend your hips.
- Relax your shoulders and neck.
- Keep your glutes tight as you bend.
- Avoid craning your neck as you perform the movement.
- Don't lift your feet off the floor.
- Avoid arching or extending your back.

MAJOR TARGETED MUSCLES
- adductor longus
- adductor magnus
- biceps femoris
- semitendinosus
- semimembranosus
- sartorius
- vastus medialis
- vastus lateralis
- vastus intermedius
- rectus femoris
- gluteus maximus
- gluteus medius
- rectus abdominis

TYPE
• Strength

TARGET
• Hips
• Knees
• Glutes
• Thighs

EQUIPMENT
• None

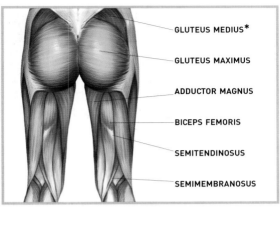

GLUTEUS MEDIUS*

GLUTEUS MAXIMUS

ADDUCTOR MAGNUS

BICEPS FEMORIS

SEMITENDINOSUS

SEMIMEMBRANOSUS

ANNOTATION KEY

BOLD = MAJOR TARGETED MUSCLES

LIGHT = SECONDARY MUSCLES

* INDICATES DEEP MUSCLES

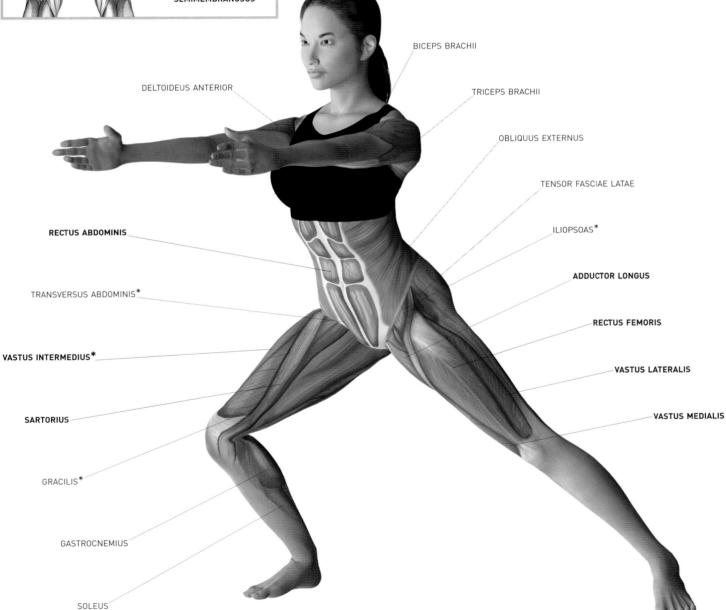

BICEPS BRACHII

DELTOIDEUS ANTERIOR

TRICEPS BRACHII

OBLIQUUS EXTERNUS

TENSOR FASCIAE LATAE

RECTUS ABDOMINIS

ILIOPSOAS*

ADDUCTOR LONGUS

TRANSVERSUS ABDOMINIS*

RECTUS FEMORIS

VASTUS INTERMEDIUS*

VASTUS LATERALIS

SARTORIUS

VASTUS MEDIALIS

GRACILIS*

GASTROCNEMIUS

SOLEUS

LATERAL-EXTENSION LATERAL LUNGE

1 Stand with your feet hip-width apart and your arms at your sides, a dumbbell in each hand.

2 Take a big step to the left, and then bend your left knee to assume a lateral lunge position. At the same time, raise both arms so that they are parallel to the floor, forming a straight line.

3 Smoothly and with control, return to the starting position.

4 Repeat on the other side, and then continue to alternate sides for a total of 10 to 12 repetitions on each leg.

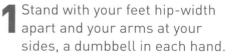

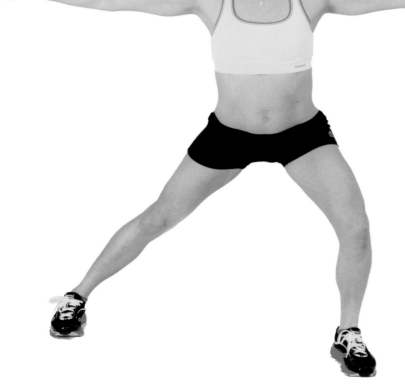

MIND YOUR FORM
- Keep your torso facing forward as you lunge to the side.
- Pull your abdominal muscles inward.
- Gaze forward.
- Avoid hunching your shoulders or arching your back.
- Avoid twisting your torso to either side.

44

TYPE
- Strength

TARGET
- Shoulders
- Legs

EQUIPMENT
- Dumbbells

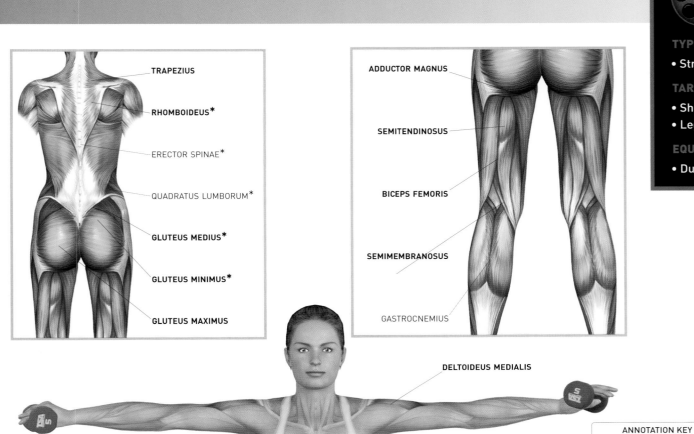

TRAPEZIUS

RHOMBOIDEUS*

ERECTOR SPINAE*

QUADRATUS LUMBORUM*

GLUTEUS MEDIUS*

GLUTEUS MINIMUS*

GLUTEUS MAXIMUS

ADDUCTOR MAGNUS

SEMITENDINOSUS

BICEPS FEMORIS

SEMIMEMBRANOSUS

GASTROCNEMIUS

DELTOIDEUS MEDIALIS

VASTUS INTERMEDIUS*

VASTUS LATERALIS

TIBIALIS ANTERIOR

ADDUCTOR LONGUS

RECTUS FEMORIS

VASTUS MEDIALIS

SOLEUS

ANNOTATION KEY

BOLD = MAJOR TARGETED MUSCLES
LIGHT = SECONDARY MUSCLES
* INDICATES DEEP MUSCLES

MAJOR TARGETED MUSCLES

- trapezius
- rhomboideus
- gluteus minimus
- gluteus medius
- gluteus maximus
- deltoideus medialis
- adductor longus
- adductor magnus
- biceps femoris
- semitendinosus
- semimembranosus
- vastus medialis
- vastus lateralis
- vastus intermedius
- rectus femoris
- gluteus maximus
- gluteus medius

WORKOUT B

Cardio-Strength Combo

Workout B builds from your strength-training experience in Workout A and then adds a vigorous cardio element. Cardiovascular exercise, also known as aerobic training, is designed to stimulate your heart rate and breathing rate. Cardio not only improves your physcial fitness, it also can elevate your mood and promote emotional health. And regular cardio offers another benefit: it helps you burn fat and build lean muscle.

4. HIGH KNEES
(Pages 48–49)

Perform two sets, alternating legs for 30 seconds.

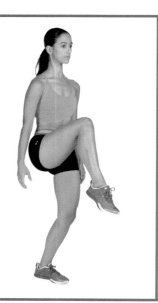

2. CHAIR ABDOMINAL CRUNCH
(Pages 50–51)

Perform two sets of 15 repetitions.

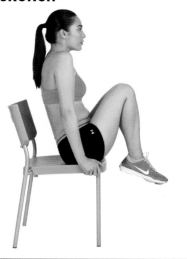

3. SPINE TWIST
(Pages 52–53)

Alternate sides for 10 repetitions on each side.

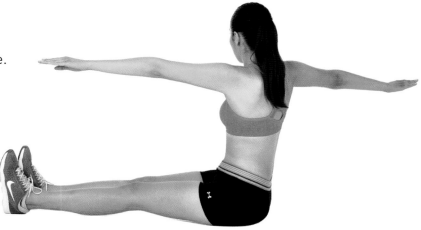

4. SWISS BALL PUSH-UP
(Pages 54–55)

Perform three sets of 10 repetitions.

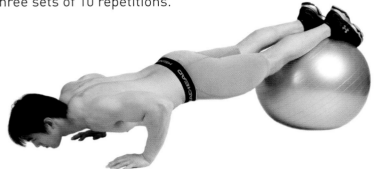

5. CURLING STEP-AND-RAISE
(Pages 56–57)

Alternate sides for 10 repetitions on each side.

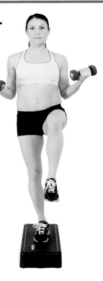

5. LATERAL STEP-DOWN
(Pages 58–59)

Perform two sets of 15 repetitions on each side.

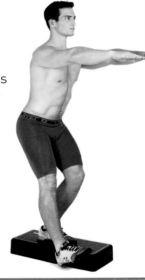

6. BUTT KICK
(Pages 60–61)

Perform for one to five minutes.

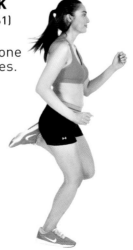

7. SHOULDER BRIDGE
(Pages 62–63)

Perform five sets, holding the pose for 30 seconds to a minute.

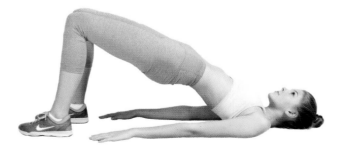

HIGH KNEES

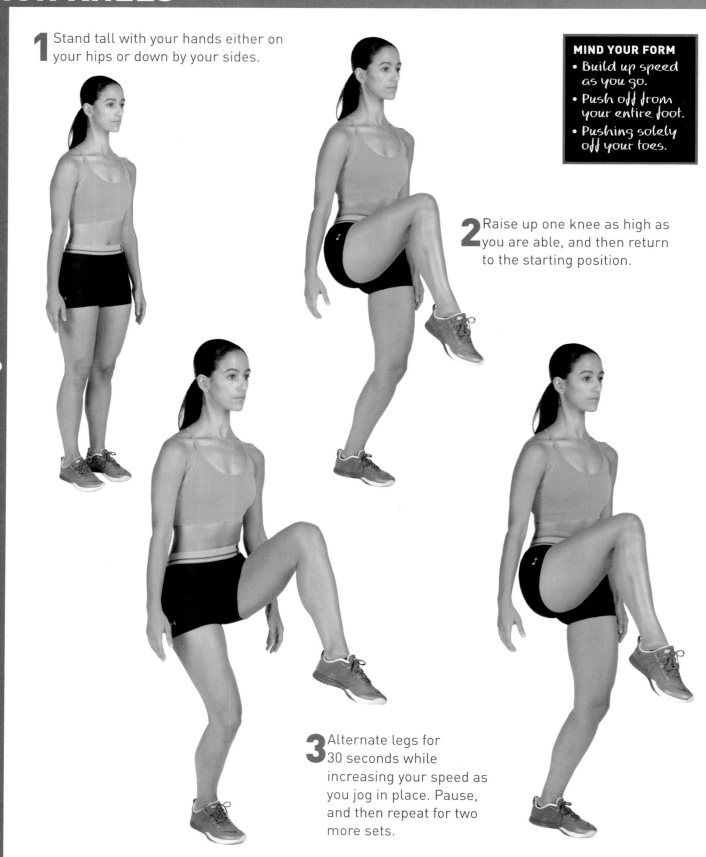

1 Stand tall with your hands either on your hips or down by your sides.

MIND YOUR FORM
- Build up speed as you go.
- Push off from your entire foot.
- Pushing solely off your toes.

2 Raise up one knee as high as you are able, and then return to the starting position.

3 Alternate legs for 30 seconds while increasing your speed as you jog in place. Pause, and then repeat for two more sets.

• Cardio

TARGET
• Legs

EQUIPMENT
• None

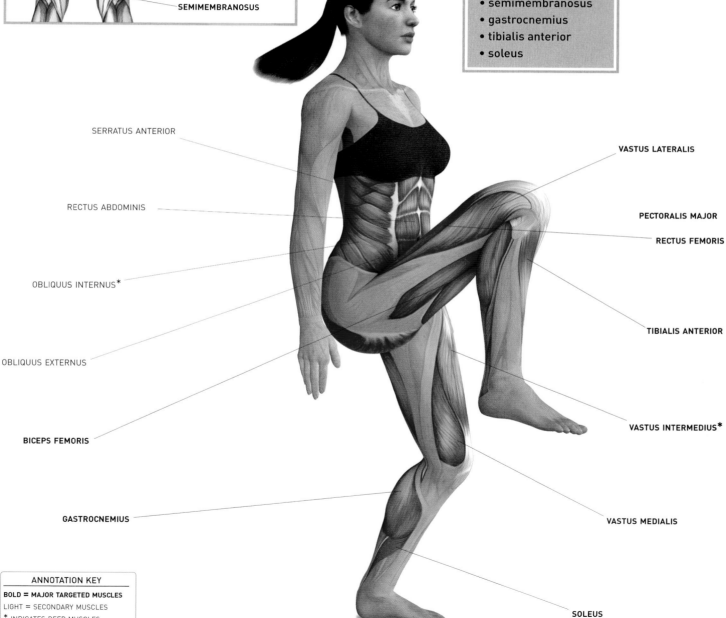

QUADRATUS LUMBORUM*
ERECTOR SPINAE*
GLUTEUS MEDIUS*
GLUTEUS MAXIMUS
PIRIFORMIS*
SEMITENDINOSUS
SEMIMEMBRANOSUS

MAJOR TARGETED MUSCLES

- gluteus maximus
- rectus femoris
- vastus lateralis
- vastus intermedius
- vastus medialis
- biceps femoris
- semitendinosus
- semimembranosus
- gastrocnemius
- tibialis anterior
- soleus

SERRATUS ANTERIOR

RECTUS ABDOMINIS

OBLIQUUS INTERNUS*

OBLIQUUS EXTERNUS

BICEPS FEMORIS

GASTROCNEMIUS

VASTUS LATERALIS

PECTORALIS MAJOR

RECTUS FEMORIS

TIBIALIS ANTERIOR

VASTUS INTERMEDIUS*

VASTUS MEDIALIS

SOLEUS

ANNOTATION KEY

BOLD = MAJOR TARGETED MUSCLES
LIGHT = SECONDARY MUSCLES
* INDICATES DEEP MUSCLES

CHAIR ABDOMINAL CRUNCH

1 Sit on a chair with your hands grasping the sides of the seat and your arms straight.

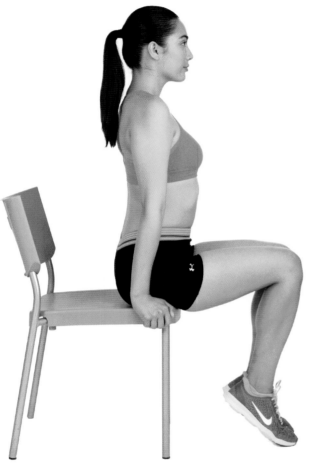

2 Tuck your torso forward and if possible lift your buttocks slightly off the chair, while swinging your legs up. Your hips and knees should be bent to form 90-degree angles.

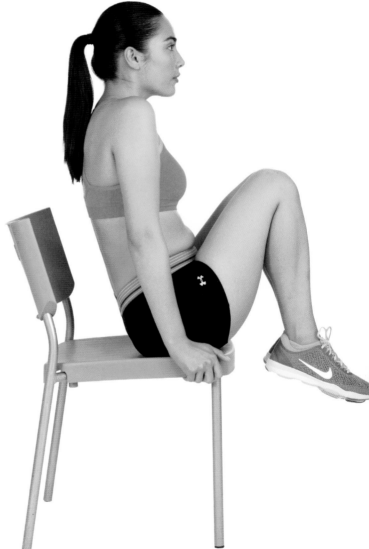

3 Tuck your tailbone toward the front of the chair, and bend your knees toward your chest. Bend your elbows simultaneously. Extend your elbows and press through your shoulders.

MIND YOUR FORM
- Make sure your spine is neutral as you progress through the motion.
- Avoid allowing your shoulders to lift up toward your ears.

4 Keeping your head in a neutral position, press into the chair and lower your legs to return to the starting position. Repeat 15 times for two sets.

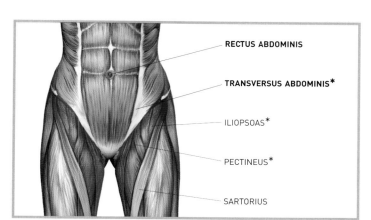

RECTUS ABDOMINIS

TRANSVERSUS ABDOMINIS*

ILIOPSOAS*

PECTINEUS*

SARTORIUS

TYPE
- Strength

TARGET
- Abdominals
- Upper arms

EQUIPMENT
- Chair

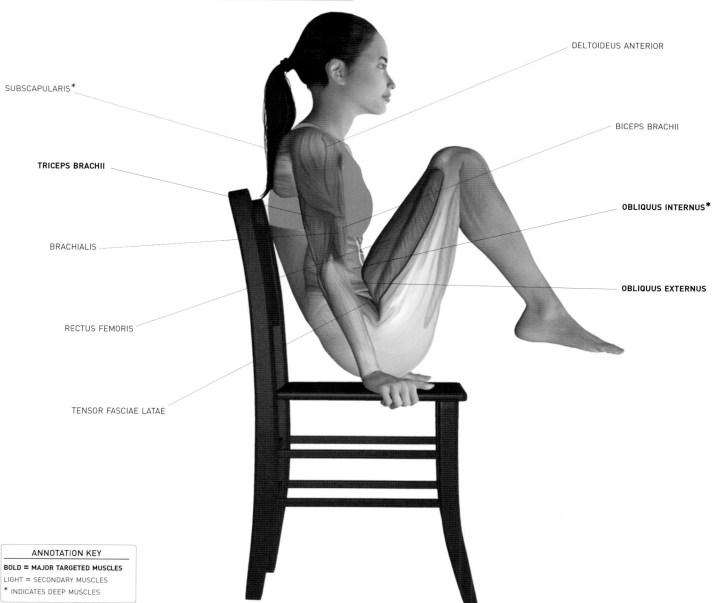

SUBSCAPULARIS*

TRICEPS BRACHII

BRACHIALIS

RECTUS FEMORIS

TENSOR FASCIAE LATAE

DELTOIDEUS ANTERIOR

BICEPS BRACHII

OBLIQUUS INTERNUS*

OBLIQUUS EXTERNUS

ANNOTATION KEY

BOLD = MAJOR TARGETED MUSCLES
LIGHT = SECONDARY MUSCLES
* INDICATES DEEP MUSCLES

SPINE TWIST

1 Sit on a mat with your legs extended and your feet slightly wider apart than your hips. Hold your back straight, and raise your arms out to the sides, fully extended, at 90 degrees to your torso.

MAJOR TARGETED MUSCLES

- deltoideus posterior
- latissimus dorsi
- gluteus maximus
- teres major
- rectus abdominis
- obliquus externus
- obliquus internus
- erector spinae
- quadratus lumborum

MIND YOUR FORM

- Keep your hips squared throughout the exercise.
- Avoid raising your hips off the floor.

2 Keeping your abdominals pulled in, twist your waist to the left, taking your entire upper body with it, then return to the central position.

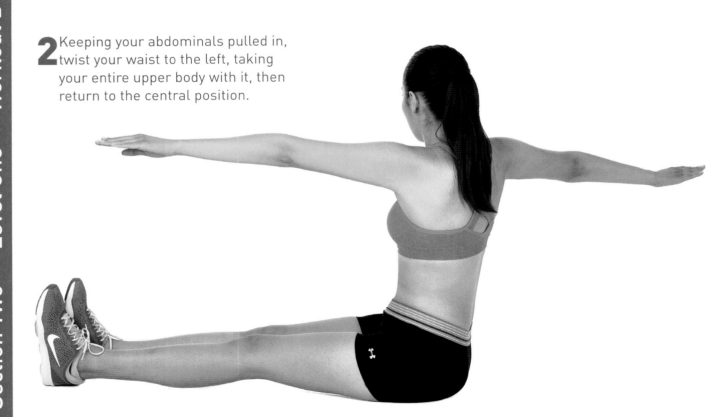

3 Repeat the movement, this time turning to the right. Complete 10 twists in each direction.

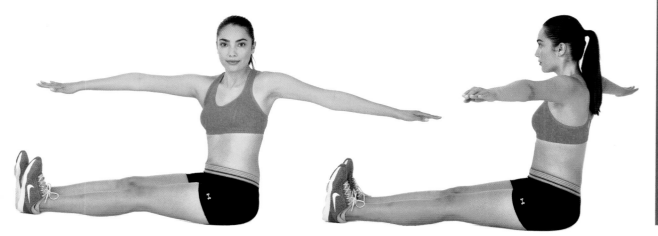

TYPE
• Strength
• Stretch

TARGET
• Back
• Abdominals
• Obliques

EQUIPMENT
• Mat

ANNOTATION KEY

BOLD = MAJOR TARGETED MUSCLES
LIGHT = SECONDARY MUSCLES
* INDICATES DEEP MUSCLES

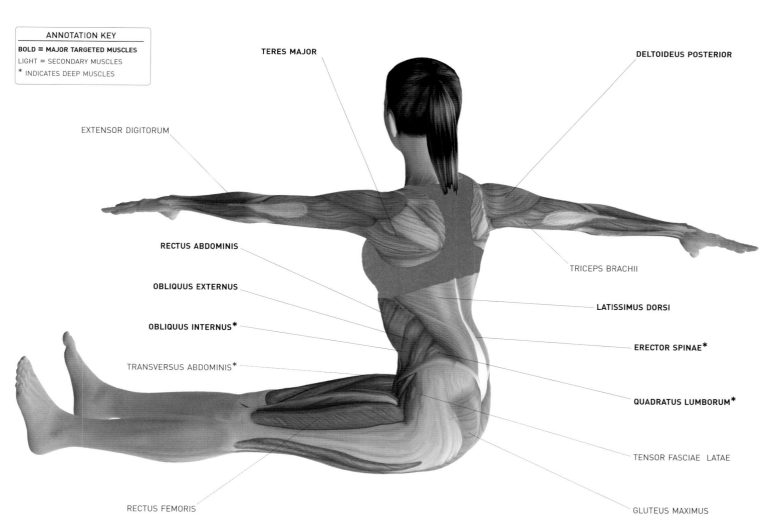

TERES MAJOR

DELTOIDEUS POSTERIOR

EXTENSOR DIGITORUM

RECTUS ABDOMINIS

TRICEPS BRACHII

OBLIQUUS EXTERNUS

LATISSIMUS DORSI

OBLIQUUS INTERNUS*

ERECTOR SPINAE*

TRANSVERSUS ABDOMINIS*

QUADRATUS LUMBORUM*

TENSOR FASCIAE LATAE

RECTUS FEMORIS

GLUTEUS MAXIMUS

SWISS BALL PUSH-UP

1 Kneel on the floor with a Swiss ball behind you. Place your toes on the point of the ball, and support your weight with your hands.

2 Walk your arms out until your legs are fully extended and your body forms a straight line from shoulders to feet, your hands shoulder-width apart.

MIND YOUR FORM
- Form a straight plane from neck to ankles.
- Inhale as you lower your torso, and exhale as you press back up.
- Avoid arching your back during the exercise.
- Don't rotate your hips.
- Don't lock your elbows.
- Avoid allowing your lower back and hips to droop – this can place increased pressure on the lumbar vertebrae and could lead to a back injury.

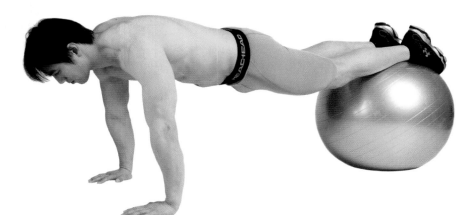

3 Lower your torso until your chest almost touches the floor.

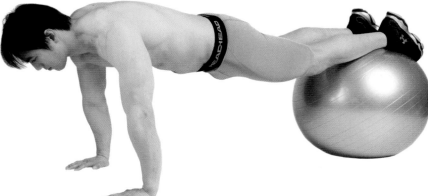

4 Press your upper body back up to the starting position, and squeeze your chest muscles. Pause at the contracted position, and repeat the raising and lowering your torso for three sets of 10 repetitions.

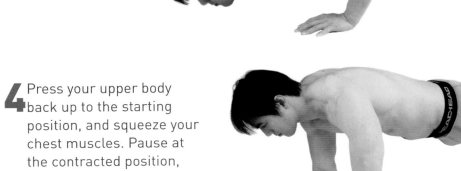

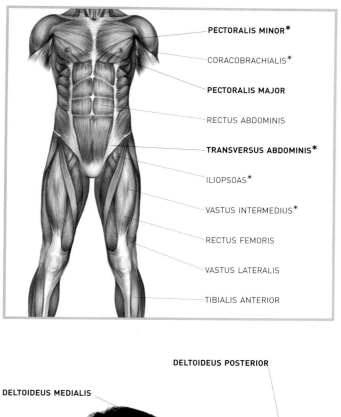

PECTORALIS MINOR*
CORACOBRACHIALIS*
PECTORALIS MAJOR
RECTUS ABDOMINIS
TRANSVERSUS ABDOMINIS*
ILIOPSOAS*
VASTUS INTERMEDIUS*
RECTUS FEMORIS
VASTUS LATERALIS
TIBIALIS ANTERIOR

MAJOR TARGETED MUSCLES

- pectoralis major
- pectoralis minor
- deltoideus posterior
- deltoideus anterior
- deltoideus medialis
- triceps brachii
- transversus abdominis
- obliquus externus
- obliquus internus

TYPE
- Strength

TARGET
- Shoulders
- Chest
- Arms

EQUIPMENT
- Swiss ball

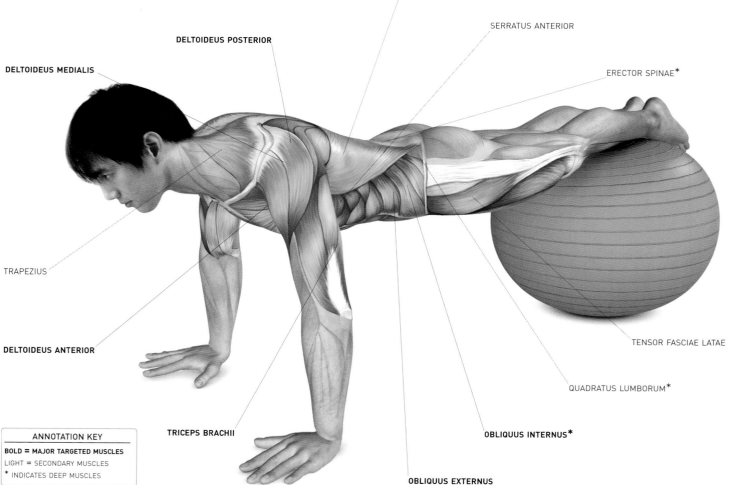

LATISSIMUS DORSI
SERRATUS ANTERIOR
ERECTOR SPINAE*
DELTOIDEUS POSTERIOR
DELTOIDEUS MEDIALIS
TRAPEZIUS
DELTOIDEUS ANTERIOR
TRICEPS BRACHII
TENSOR FASCIAE LATAE
QUADRATUS LUMBORUM*
OBLIQUUS INTERNUS*
OBLIQUUS EXTERNUS

ANNOTATION KEY

BOLD = MAJOR TARGETED MUSCLES
LIGHT = SECONDARY MUSCLES
* INDICATES DEEP MUSCLES

CURLING STEP-AND-RAISE

1 Stand with your feet hip-width apart and your arms at your sides, a dumbbell in each hand. Position a step beside your left foot.

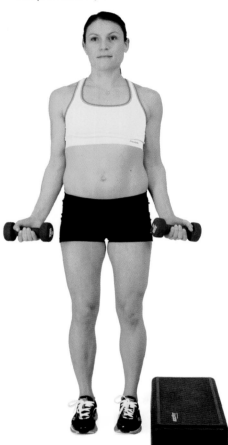

2 Place your left foot on the step.

3 Shift your weight onto your left foot. Bend your elbows, curling the dumbbells toward your chest. At the same time, raise your right knee as the foot comes off the floor. Continue raising and curling until your right leg forms a right angle and your dumbbells are nearly at shoulder height.

MIND YOUR FORM
- Keep your upper arms stationary as you curl and release.
- Keep your movements smooth and controlled.
- Keep your torso facing forward.
- Pull your abdominal muscles inward.
- Gaze forward.
- Press your shoulders away from your ears.

4 Lower the dumbbells, cross your right leg over your left leg, which should bend slightly as you lower your right leg to the floor, left of the platform. Simultaneously bend your left leg slightly.

5 Step your left leg onto the floor so that you are in starting position on the other side of the step.

6 Repeat on the other side. Continue to alternate sides, aiming for 20 repetitions.

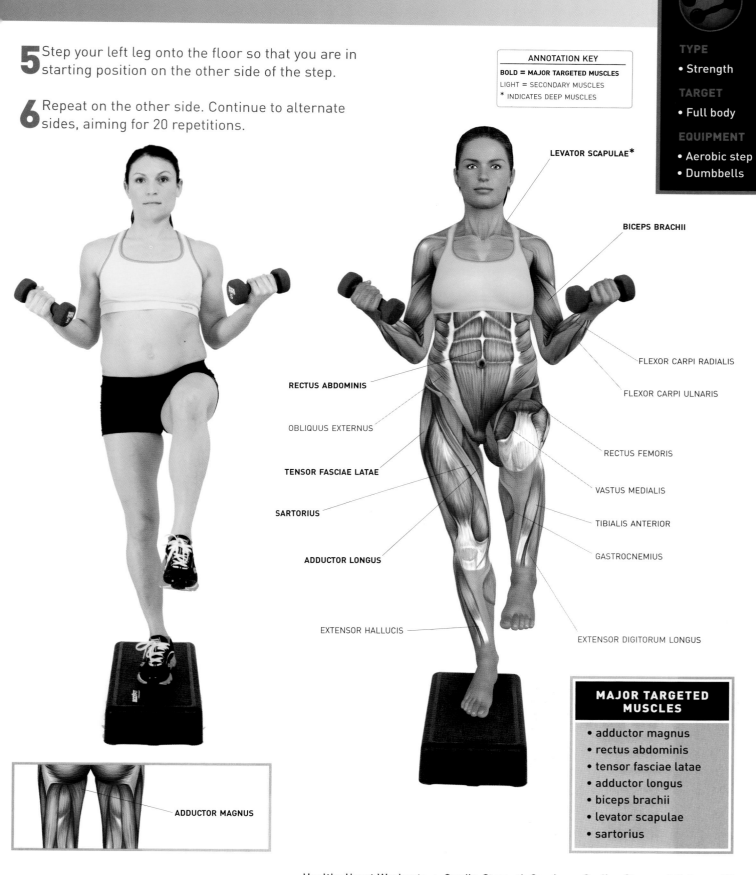

ANNOTATION KEY

BOLD = MAJOR TARGETED MUSCLES
LIGHT = SECONDARY MUSCLES
* INDICATES DEEP MUSCLES

TYPE
• Strength

TARGET
• Full body

EQUIPMENT
• Aerobic step
• Dumbbells

LEVATOR SCAPULAE*

BICEPS BRACHII

FLEXOR CARPI RADIALIS

FLEXOR CARPI ULNARIS

RECTUS ABDOMINIS

OBLIQUUS EXTERNUS

RECTUS FEMORIS

TENSOR FASCIAE LATAE

VASTUS MEDIALIS

SARTORIUS

TIBIALIS ANTERIOR

GASTROCNEMIUS

ADDUCTOR LONGUS

EXTENSOR HALLUCIS

EXTENSOR DIGITORUM LONGUS

ADDUCTOR MAGNUS

MAJOR TARGETED MUSCLES

• adductor magnus
• rectus abdominis
• tensor fasciae latae
• adductor longus
• biceps brachii
• levator scapulae
• sartorius

LATERAL STEP-DOWN

1 Standing up straight on a firm step or block, plant your left foot firmly close to the edge, and allow your right foot to hang off the side. Flex the toes of your right foot.

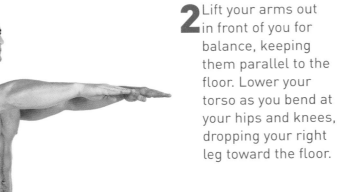

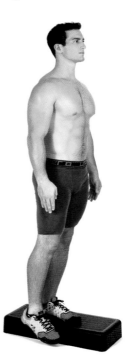

2 Lift your arms out in front of you for balance, keeping them parallel to the floor. Lower your torso as you bend at your hips and knees, dropping your right leg toward the floor.

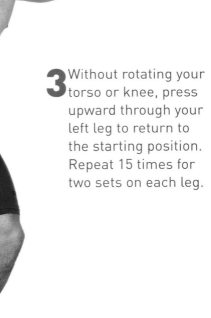

3 Without rotating your torso or knee, press upward through your left leg to return to the starting position. Repeat 15 times for two sets on each leg.

MIND YOUR FORM
- Align your bent knee with your second toe so that your knee doesn't rotate inward.
- Bend your knees and hips at the same time.
- Keep your hips behind your foot, leaning your torso forward as you lower into the bend.
- Avoid craning your neck.
- Avoid placing weight on the foot being lowered to the floor—only allow a slight touch.

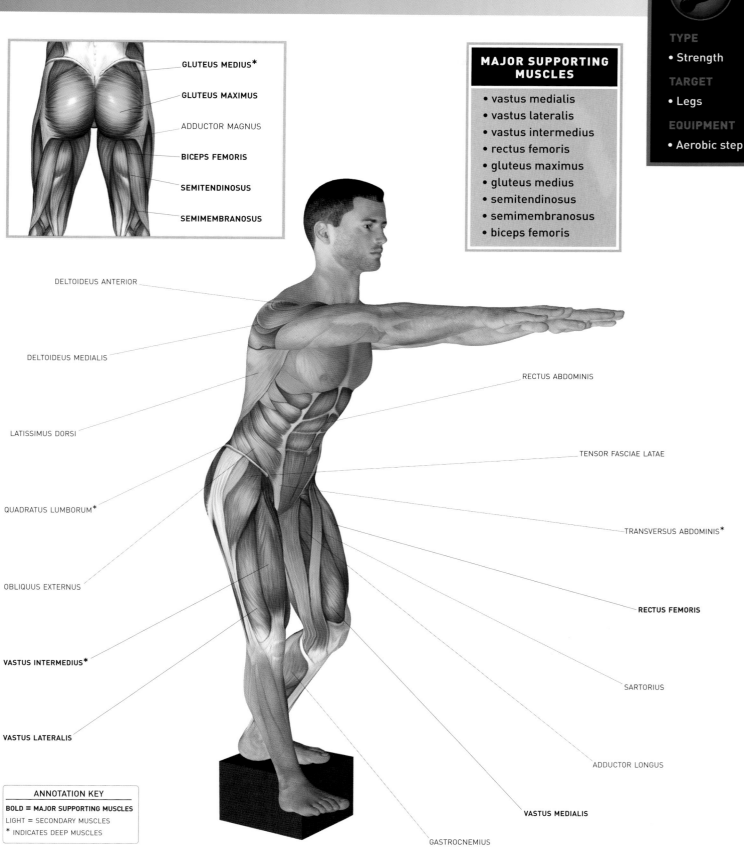

GLUTEUS MEDIUS*

GLUTEUS MAXIMUS

ADDUCTOR MAGNUS

BICEPS FEMORIS

SEMITENDINOSUS

SEMIMEMBRANOSUS

MAJOR SUPPORTING MUSCLES

- vastus medialis
- vastus lateralis
- vastus intermedius
- rectus femoris
- gluteus maximus
- gluteus medius
- semitendinosus
- semimembranosus
- biceps femoris

TYPE
- Strength

TARGET
- Legs

EQUIPMENT
- Aerobic step

DELTOIDEUS ANTERIOR

DELTOIDEUS MEDIALIS

LATISSIMUS DORSI

QUADRATUS LUMBORUM*

OBLIQUUS EXTERNUS

VASTUS INTERMEDIUS*

VASTUS LATERALIS

RECTUS ABDOMINIS

TENSOR FASCIAE LATAE

TRANSVERSUS ABDOMINIS*

RECTUS FEMORIS

SARTORIUS

ADDUCTOR LONGUS

VASTUS MEDIALIS

GASTROCNEMIUS

ANNOTATION KEY

BOLD = MAJOR SUPPORTING MUSCLES
LIGHT = SECONDARY MUSCLES
* INDICATES DEEP MUSCLES

BUTT KICK

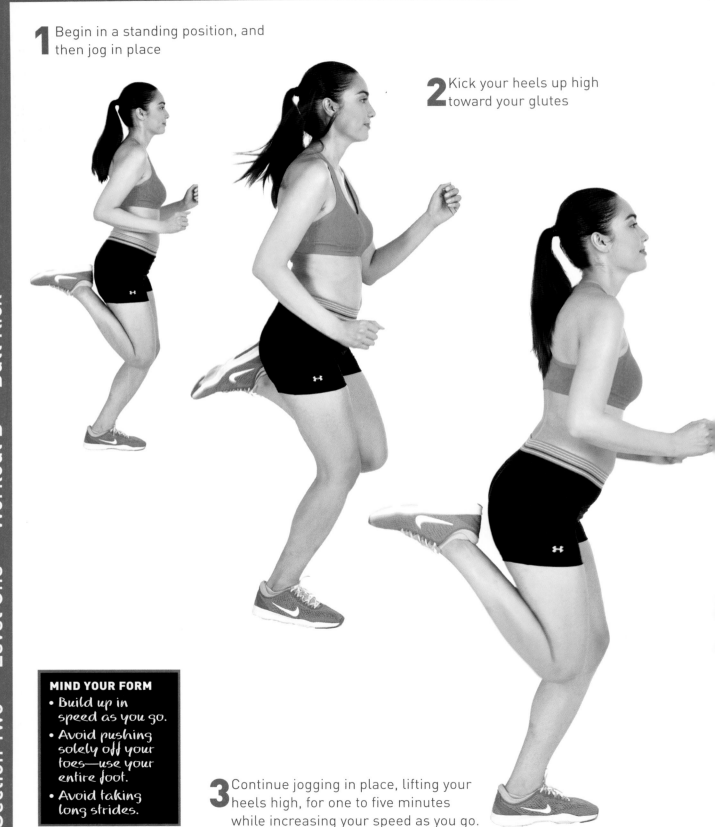

1 Begin in a standing position, and then jog in place

2 Kick your heels up high toward your glutes

MIND YOUR FORM
- Build up in speed as you go.
- Avoid pushing solely off your toes—use your entire foot.
- Avoid taking long strides.

3 Continue jogging in place, lifting your heels high, for one to five minutes while increasing your speed as you go.

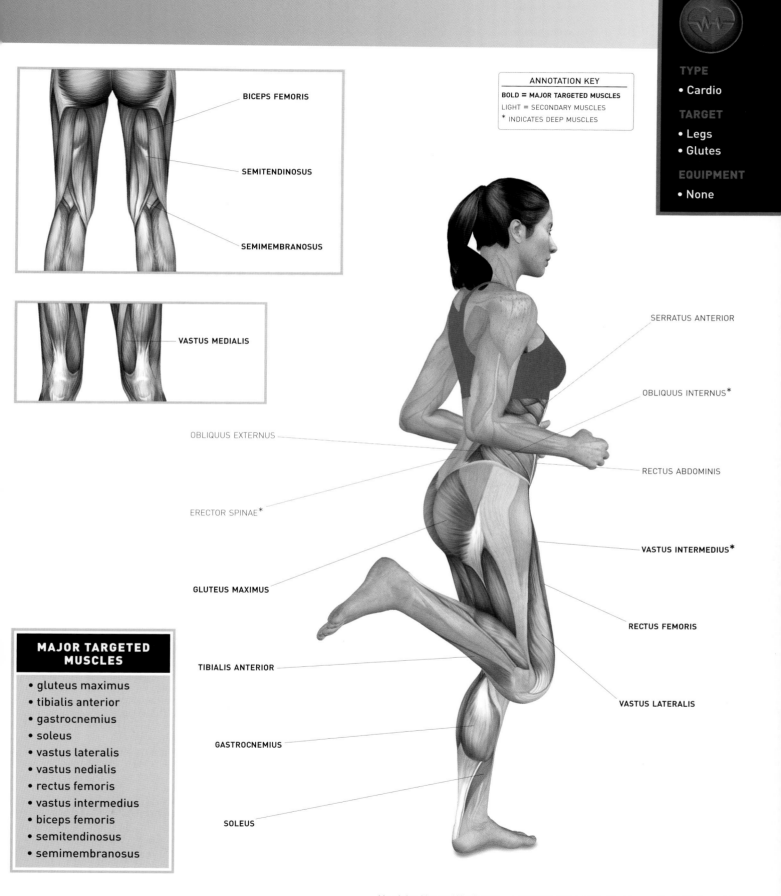

BICEPS FEMORIS

SEMITENDINOSUS

SEMIMEMBRANOSUS

VASTUS MEDIALIS

ANNOTATION KEY

BOLD = MAJOR TARGETED MUSCLES
LIGHT = SECONDARY MUSCLES
* INDICATES DEEP MUSCLES

SERRATUS ANTERIOR

OBLIQUUS INTERNUS*

OBLIQUUS EXTERNUS

RECTUS ABDOMINIS

ERECTOR SPINAE*

VASTUS INTERMEDIUS*

GLUTEUS MAXIMUS

RECTUS FEMORIS

TIBIALIS ANTERIOR

VASTUS LATERALIS

GASTROCNEMIUS

SOLEUS

MAJOR TARGETED MUSCLES

• gluteus maximus
• tibialis anterior
• gastrocnemius
• soleus
• vastus lateralis
• vastus nedialis
• rectus femoris
• vastus intermedius
• biceps femoris
• semitendinosus
• semimembranosus

SHOULDER BRIDGE

1 Lie faceup on a mat with your legs bent, your feet flat on the floor, and your arms extended at your sides, angled slightly away from your body.

MIND YOUR FORM
- Push through your heels, not your toes.
- Keep your knees and feet aligned.
- Keep your arms and feet on the floor.
- Avoid overextending your abdominals past your thighs in the finished position.
- Avoid arching your back or letting your torso sag.

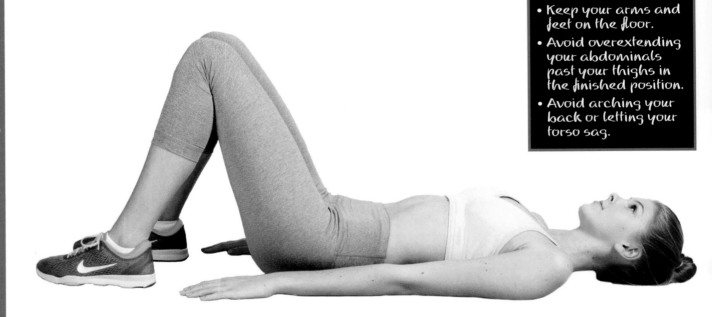

2 Push through your heels while raising your pelvis until your torso is aligned with your thighs. Hold for 30 seconds to a minute, and then lower your pelvis to the starting position. Repeat for five repetitions.

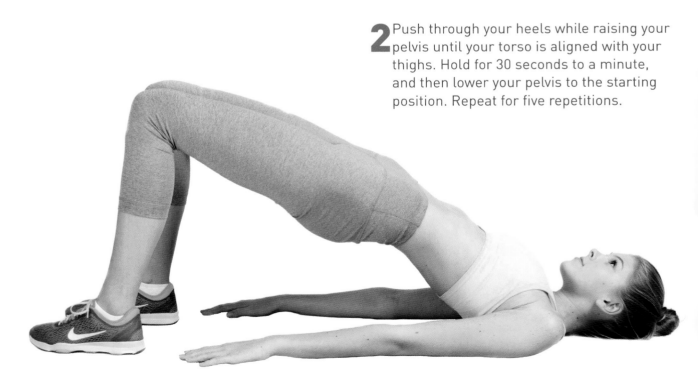

TYPE
• Strength
TARGET
• Full body
EQUIPMENT
• Mat

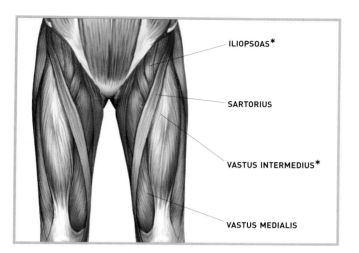

ILIOPSOAS*

SARTORIUS

VASTUS INTERMEDIUS*

VASTUS MEDIALIS

MAJOR TARGETED MUSCLES

• erector spinae
• iliopsoas
• sartorius
• rectus femoris
• gluteus maximus
• gluteus medius
• gluteus minimus
• vastus lateralis
• vastus intermedius
• vastus medialis

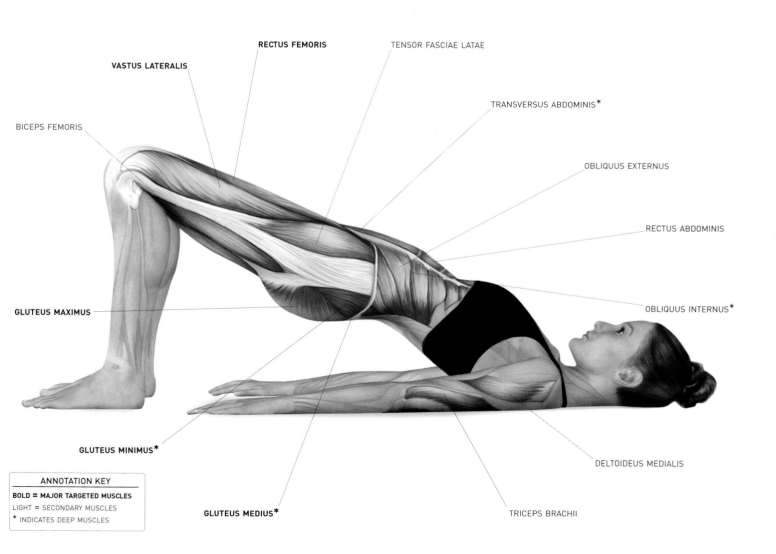

RECTUS FEMORIS

TENSOR FASCIAE LATAE

VASTUS LATERALIS

TRANSVERSUS ABDOMINIS*

BICEPS FEMORIS

OBLIQUUS EXTERNUS

RECTUS ABDOMINIS

GLUTEUS MAXIMUS

OBLIQUUS INTERNUS*

GLUTEUS MINIMUS*

DELTOIDEUS MEDIALIS

ANNOTATION KEY

BOLD = MAJOR TARGETED MUSCLES
LIGHT = SECONDARY MUSCLES
* INDICATES DEEP MUSCLES

GLUTEUS MEDIUS*

TRICEPS BRACHII

Level One

WORKOUT C

Full-Body Stretch Sequence

Stretches and other flexibility exercises are key elements in a Healthy Heart workout regimen. Long a staple of exercise warm-ups, stretching moves have now been switched from the start of a workout to the end. Try this beginner-level stretching routine to help counteract any post-workout muscle tightness, especially in your back.

1. SKATER'S LUNGE
(Pages 66–67)

Perform 25 repetitions.

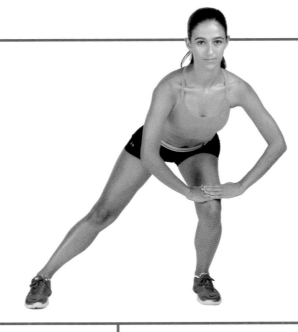

2. SIDE BEND
(Pages 68–69)

Perform the entire sequence five times.

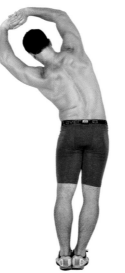

3. LATISSIMUS DORSI STRETCH
(Pages 70–71)

Perform the entire sequence three times in each direction

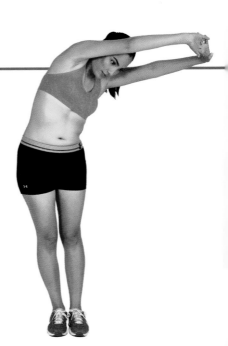

4. DIAGONAL REACH
(Pages 72–73)

Alternate sides for 10 repetitions on each side.

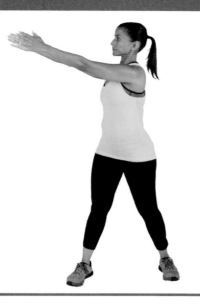

5. ILIOTIBIAL BAND STRETCH
(Pages 74–75)

Perform one repetition on each side, holding the stretch for 20 seconds.

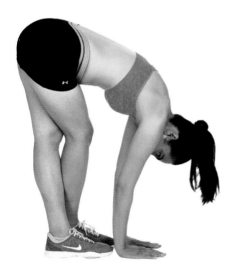

3. SIDE-LYING KNEE BEND
(Pages 76–77)

Perform one repetition on each side, holding the stretch for 20 seconds.

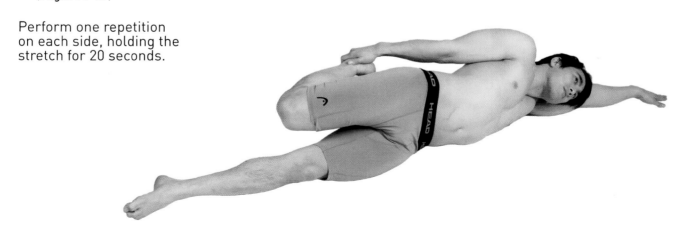

SKATER'S LUNGE

1 Stand with your legs spaced wider than shoulder-width apart and your toes pointing forward.

2 Slide to your side into a lateral lunge as you bend forward slightly, placing your hands on your bent knee.

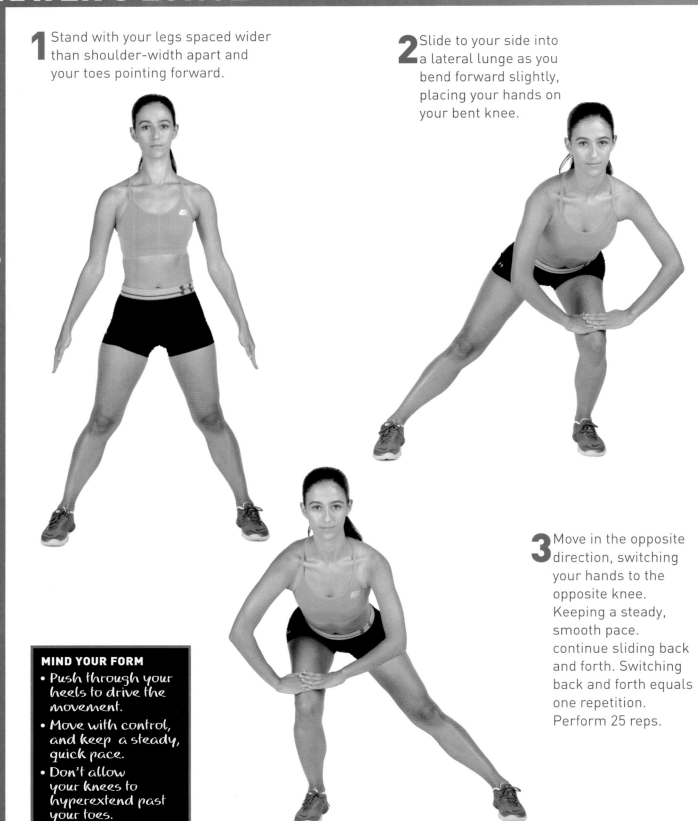

3 Move in the opposite direction, switching your hands to the opposite knee. Keeping a steady, smooth pace. continue sliding back and forth. Switching back and forth equals one repetition. Perform 25 reps.

MIND YOUR FORM
- Push through your heels to drive the movement.
- Move with control, and keep a steady, quick pace.
- Don't allow your knees to hyperextend past your toes.

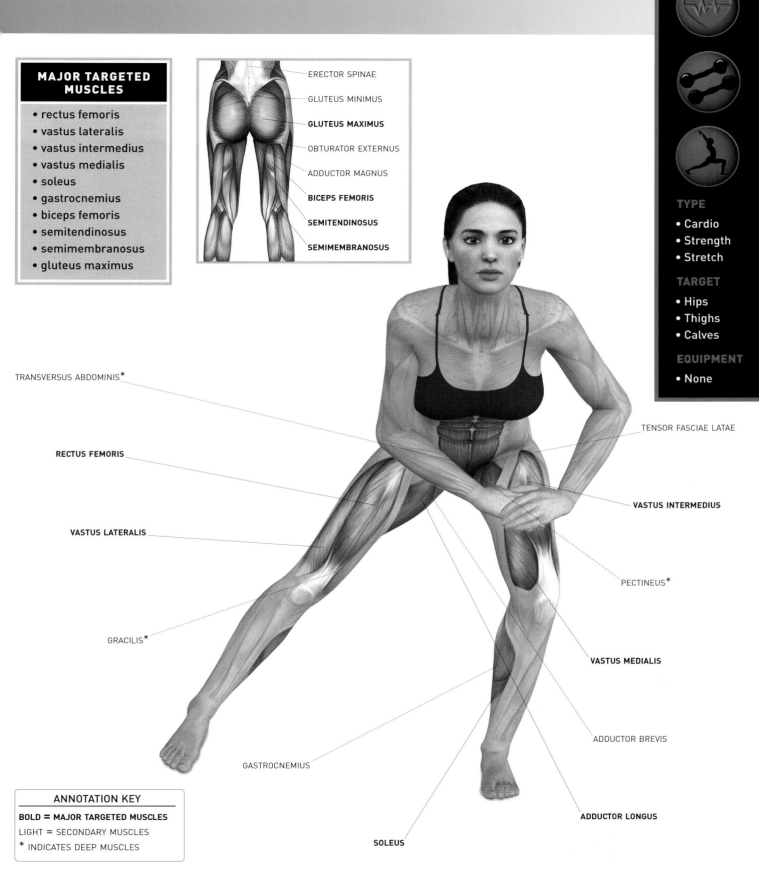

MAJOR TARGETED MUSCLES

- rectus femoris
- vastus lateralis
- vastus intermedius
- vastus medialis
- soleus
- gastrocnemius
- biceps femoris
- semitendinosus
- semimembranosus
- gluteus maximus

ERECTOR SPINAE

GLUTEUS MINIMUS

GLUTEUS MAXIMUS

OBTURATOR EXTERNUS

ADDUCTOR MAGNUS

BICEPS FEMORIS

SEMITENDINOSUS

SEMIMEMBRANOSUS

TYPE
- Cardio
- Strength
- Stretch

TARGET
- Hips
- Thighs
- Calves

EQUIPMENT
- None

TRANSVERSUS ABDOMINIS*

RECTUS FEMORIS

VASTUS LATERALIS

GRACILIS*

TENSOR FASCIAE LATAE

VASTUS INTERMEDIUS

PECTINEUS*

VASTUS MEDIALIS

ADDUCTOR BREVIS

GASTROCNEMIUS

ADDUCTOR LONGUS

SOLEUS

ANNOTATION KEY

BOLD = MAJOR TARGETED MUSCLES

LIGHT = SECONDARY MUSCLES

* INDICATES DEEP MUSCLES

SIDE BEND

1 Stand, keeping your neck, shoulders, and torso straight.

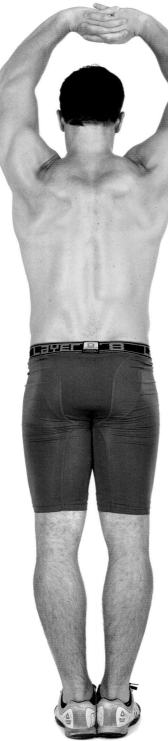

2 Raise both arms above your head and clasp your hands together, palms facing upward.

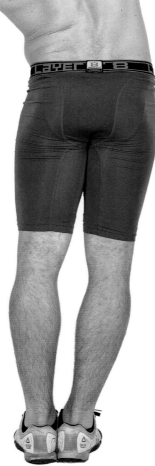

3 Leaning from the hips, slowly drop your torso to the left.

TYPE
• Stretch
TARGET
• Back
EQUIPMENT
• None

MAJOR TARGETED MUSCLES

- latissimus dorsi
- erector spinae
- obliquus externus
- obliquus internus
- teres major
- teres minor

ANNOTATION KEY

BOLD = MAJOR TARGETED MUSCLES
LIGHT = SECONDARY MUSCLES
* INDICATES DEEP MUSCLES

DELTOIDEUS POSTERIOR

TRAPEZIUS

TERES MINOR

TERES MAJOR

LATISSIMUS DORSI

ERECTOR SPINAE*

4 Keeping a smooth flow, lean your torso to the right. Repeat the entire sequence five times.

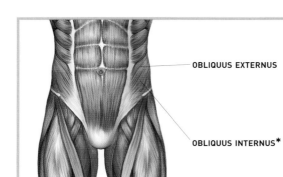

OBLIQUUS EXTERNUS

OBLIQUUS INTERNUS*

LATISSIMUS DORSI STRETCH

1 Stand, keeping your neck, shoulders, and torso straight.

2 Raise both arms above your head and clasp your hands together, palms facing upward.

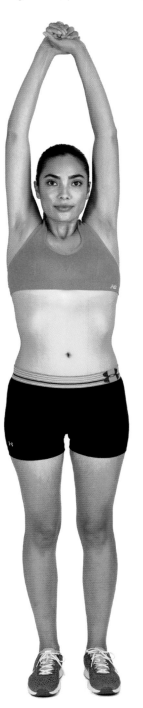

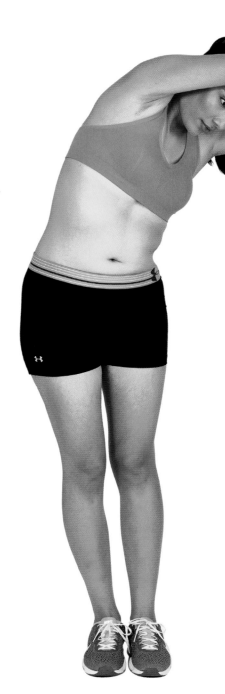

3 Keeping your elbows straight, reach to the side to begin tracing a circular pattern with your torso

4 Lean forward and then to the opposite side as you slowly trace a full circle.

5 Return to the starting position, and then repeat the sequence three times in each direction.

TYPE
• Stretch

TARGET
• Back
• Shoulder
• Obliques

EQUIPMENT
• None

ANNOTATION KEY

BOLD = MAJOR TARGETED MUSCLES
LIGHT = SECONDARY MUSCLES
* INDICATES DEEP MUSCLES

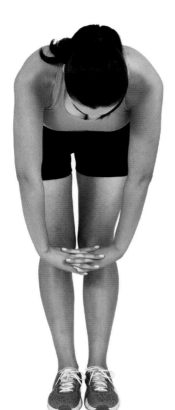

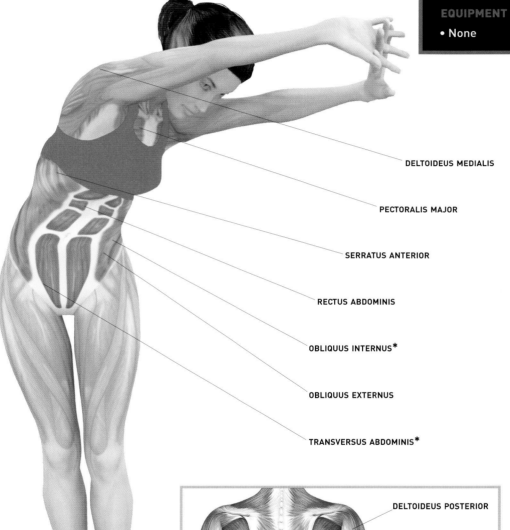

DELTOIDEUS MEDIALIS

PECTORALIS MAJOR

SERRATUS ANTERIOR

RECTUS ABDOMINIS

OBLIQUUS INTERNUS*

OBLIQUUS EXTERNUS

TRANSVERSUS ABDOMINIS*

DELTOIDEUS POSTERIOR

TRAPEZIUS

TERES MINOR

TERES MAJOR

LATISSIMUS DORSI

MAJOR TARGETED MUSCLES

• deltoideus medialis
• deltoideus posterior
• pectoralis major
• serratus anterior
• obliquus internus
• obliquus externus
• rectus abdominis
• transversus abdominis
• latissimus dorsi
• trapezius

DIAGONAL REACH

1 Stand with your feet hip-width apart and your arms at your sides.

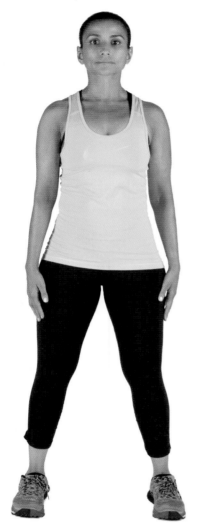

2 Raise both arms upward and to the right to form a diagonal line. Follow your hands with your gaze.

3 Return to starting position, and then repeat to the left side. Continue alternating sides for a total of 10 repetitions to each side.

MIND YOUR FORM
• Keep your abdominal muscles engaged throughout the movement keeping your hips facing forward and your shoulders pressed down. Avoid twisting your hips, hunching your shoulders, or tensing your neck as you lift or lower your arms.

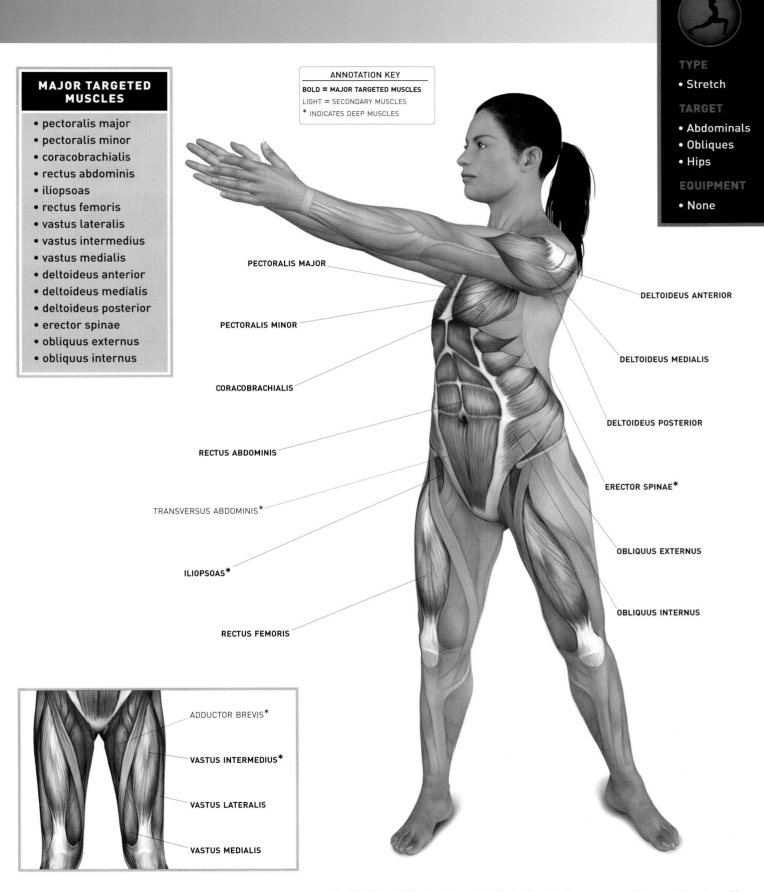

MAJOR TARGETED MUSCLES

- pectoralis major
- pectoralis minor
- coracobrachialis
- rectus abdominis
- iliopsoas
- rectus femoris
- vastus lateralis
- vastus intermedius
- vastus medialis
- deltoideus anterior
- deltoideus medialis
- deltoideus posterior
- erector spinae
- obliquus externus
- obliquus internus

ANNOTATION KEY

BOLD = MAJOR TARGETED MUSCLES
LIGHT = SECONDARY MUSCLES
* INDICATES DEEP MUSCLES

TYPE
- Stretch

TARGET
- Abdominals
- Obliques
- Hips

EQUIPMENT
- None

PECTORALIS MAJOR

PECTORALIS MINOR

CORACOBRACHIALIS

RECTUS ABDOMINIS

TRANSVERSUS ABDOMINIS*

ILIOPSOAS*

RECTUS FEMORIS

DELTOIDEUS ANTERIOR

DELTOIDEUS MEDIALIS

DELTOIDEUS POSTERIOR

ERECTOR SPINAE*

OBLIQUUS EXTERNUS

OBLIQUUS INTERNUS

ADDUCTOR BREVIS*

VASTUS INTERMEDIUS*

VASTUS LATERALIS

VASTUS MEDIALIS

ILIOTIBIAL BAND STRETCH

1 Start in a standing position, and cross your left foot behind the right ankle.

MIND YOUR FORM
- Slowly ease into the movement: never force a stretch.
- Avoid overextending your legs.
- If you can't at first touch the floor, bend forward and place your hand on your knees.

2 Lean forward until you are as close to the floor with your fingertips as you can go. If you are able, grasp your toes, or, as a more difficult modification, place your hands flat on the floor.

3 Hold for 20 seconds and repeat, then switch legs and repeat the entire stretch.

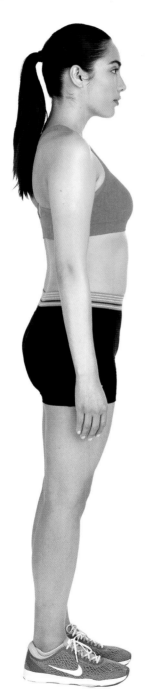

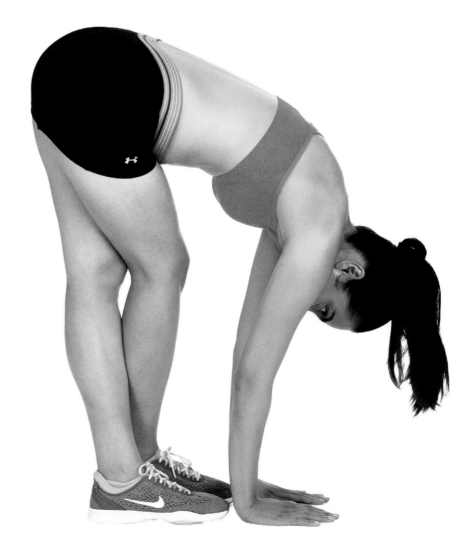

TYPE
• Stretch

TARGET
• Hamstrings
• Iliotibial band

EQUIPMENT
• None

GLUTEUS MEDIUS*

GLUTEUS MINIMUS

OBTURATOR EXTERNUS

SEMITENDINOSUS

SEMIMEMBRANOSUS

MAJOR TARGETED MUSCLES

- gluteus maximus
- tractus iliotibialis
- vastus lateralis
- rectus femoris
- semitendinosus
- semimembranosus
- biceps femoris

GLUTEUS MAXIMUS

TRACTUS ILIOTIBIALIS

BICEPS FEMORIS

VASTUS LATERALIS

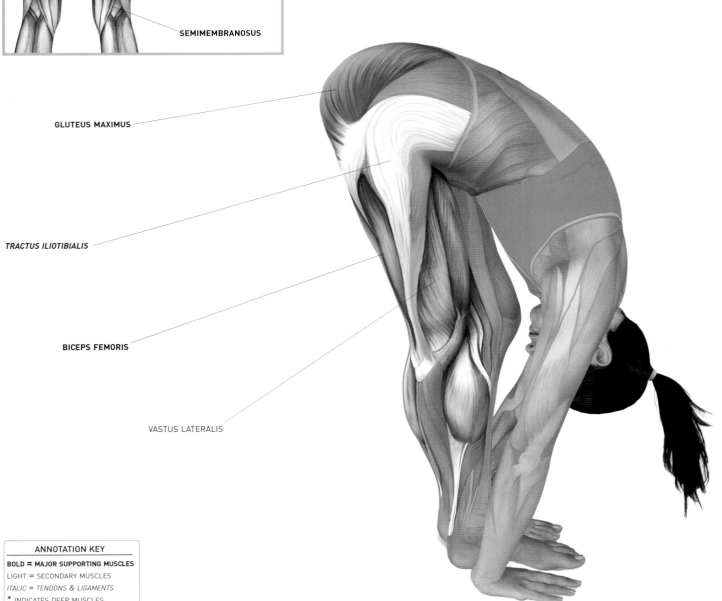

ANNOTATION KEY

BOLD = MAJOR SUPPORTING MUSCLES
LIGHT = SECONDARY MUSCLES
ITALIC = TENDONS & LIGAMENTS
* INDICATES DEEP MUSCLES

SIDE-LYING KNEE BEND

1 Lie on on a mat on your left side, with your legs extended together in line with your body. Extend your left arm, and rest your head on your upper arm.

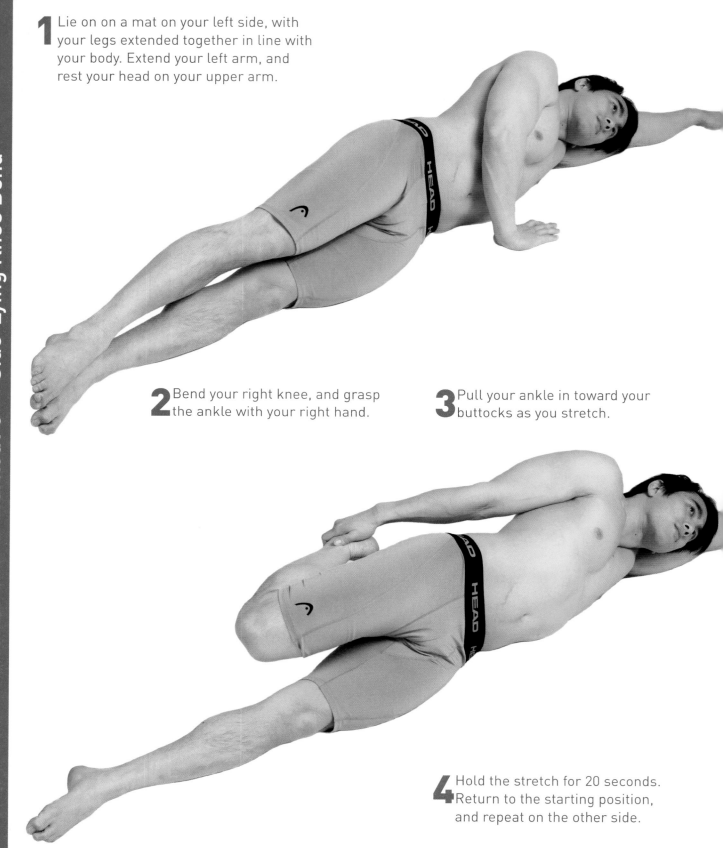

2 Bend your right knee, and grasp the ankle with your right hand.

3 Pull your ankle in toward your buttocks as you stretch.

4 Hold the stretch for 20 seconds. Return to the starting position, and repeat on the other side.

MIND YOUR FORM

- Keep your knees together, one on top of the other.
- Tuck your pelvis slightly forward and lift your chest to engage and stretch your core.
- Keep your foot pointed and parallel with your leg.
- Avoid leaning back onto your gluteal muscles.
- Place a towel under your bottom hip if it feels uncomfortable to rest directly on the floor.

MAJOR TARGETED MUSCLES

- rectus femoris
- vastus lateralis
- vastus intermedius
- vastus medialis

TYPE
- Stretch

TARGET
- Thighs

EQUIPMENT
- Mat

ANNOTATION KEY

BOLD = MAJOR TARGETED MUSCLES
LIGHT = SECONDARY MUSCLES
* INDICATES DEEP MUSCLES

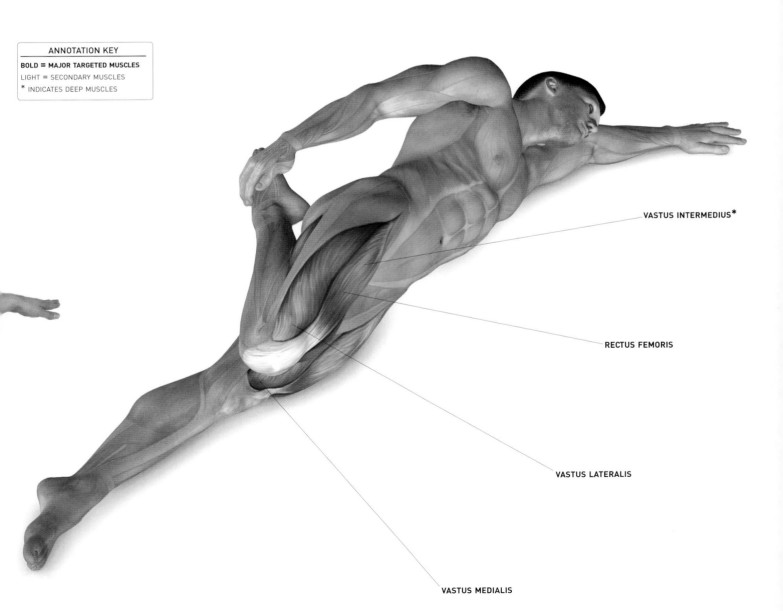

VASTUS INTERMEDIUS*

RECTUS FEMORIS

VASTUS LATERALIS

VASTUS MEDIALIS

LEVEL TWO

Once you have developed basic strength, flexibility, and stamina by mastering the workouts in Level One, it is time to take that progress a bit further. Level Two workouts will challenge you to go beyond your previous efforts, calling for you to perform more complex exercises in longer workouts that really get your heart pumping, while continuing to help you to build lean muscle.

As you master the exercises in this section and continue to practice what you learned in Level One, periodically check back to this page to see how are progressing toward the goals listed in the chart below. Once you have safely achieved all these milestones, you can move on to the workouts shown in Level Three.

LEVEL TWO PROGRESS REPORT

WORKOUT	NAME	GOAL
A	Strength and Stamina Sequence	Improve full-body muscle strength and increase stamina and endurance
B	Core and Balance Sequence	Build abdominal strength and improve balance and coordination.

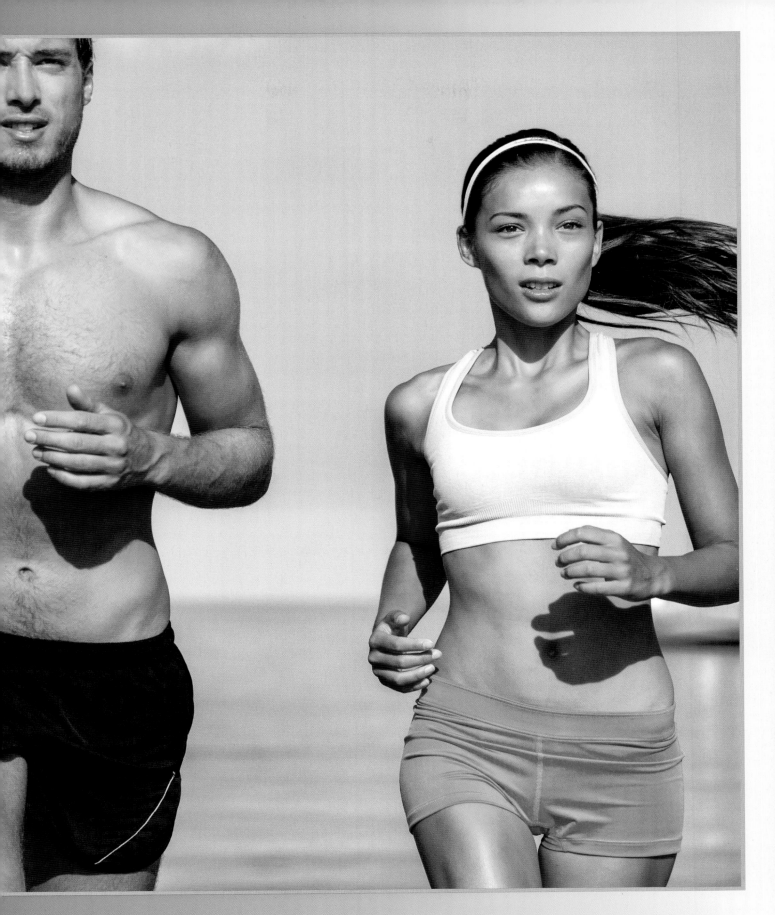

WORKOUT A

Strength and Stamina Sequence

Start your joint health regimen at the top, with a workout that targets your neck and shoulders. Whether you spend hours at your desk peering at a computer screen or toss heavy weights like a book-laden backpack across your shoulders every day, this area can too often hold a lot of tension. Try this beginner-level workout to help counteract that tightness and keep your shoulder and neck joints moving smoothly.

1. POWER PUNCH
(Pages 82–83)

Perform three sets of 10 repetitions on each side.

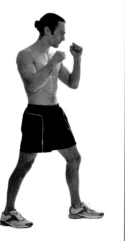

2. STAR JUMP
(Pages 84–85)

Perform 15 to 20 repetitions.

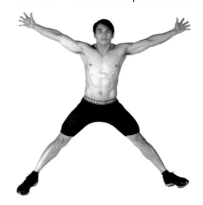

3. LATERAL BOUNDING
(Pages xx–xx7)

Perform for one to five minutes.

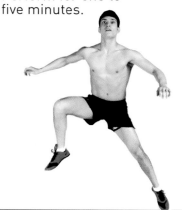

4. WALKING LUNGE
(Pages 86–87)

Perform 25 repetitions on each side.

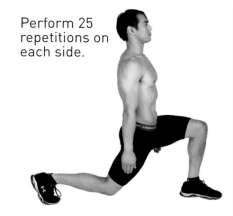

5. LEG-EXTENSION CHAIR DIP
(Pages88–89)

Perform 10 repetitions on each side.

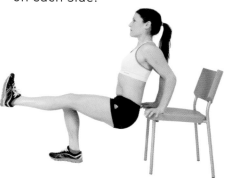

6. SINGLE-LEG CIRCLES
(Pages 90–91)

Perform 10 repetitions on each side.

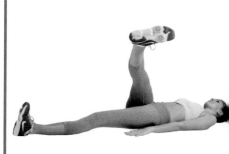

7. ROLL-UP TRICEPS LIFT
(Pages 92–93)

Perform 10 repetitions.

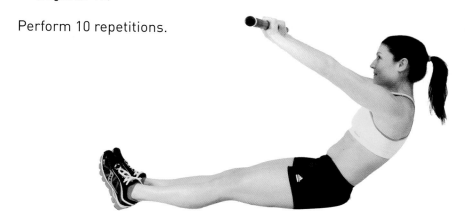

EQUIPMENT CHECKLIST
- ✘ Swiss ball
- ✔ medicine ball
- ✘ dumbbells
- ✔ barbell
- ✘ kettlebells
- ✔ mat
- ✔ chair
- ✘ bench
- ✔ aerobic step
- ✘ towel

8. SEATED RUSSIAN TWIST
(Pages 94–95)

Perform 20 repetitions on each side.

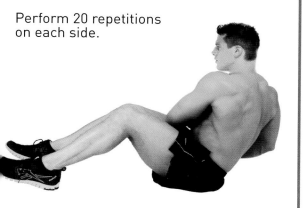

9. BEAR CRAWL
(Pages 96–97)

Perform for one to five minutes.

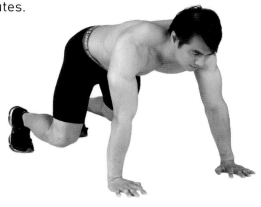

10. CROSSOVER STEP-UP
(Pages 98–99)

Perform 15 repetitions on each side.

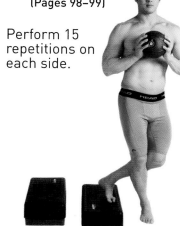

11. POWER SQUAT
(Pages 100–101)

Perform two sets of 15 repetitions on each side.

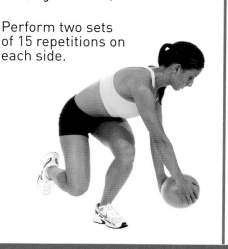

12. HIP-TO THIGH STRETCH
(Pages102–103)

Perform five repetitions on each side.

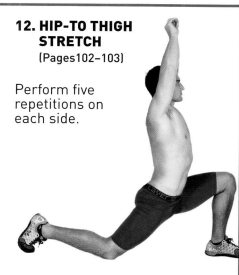

POWER PUNCH

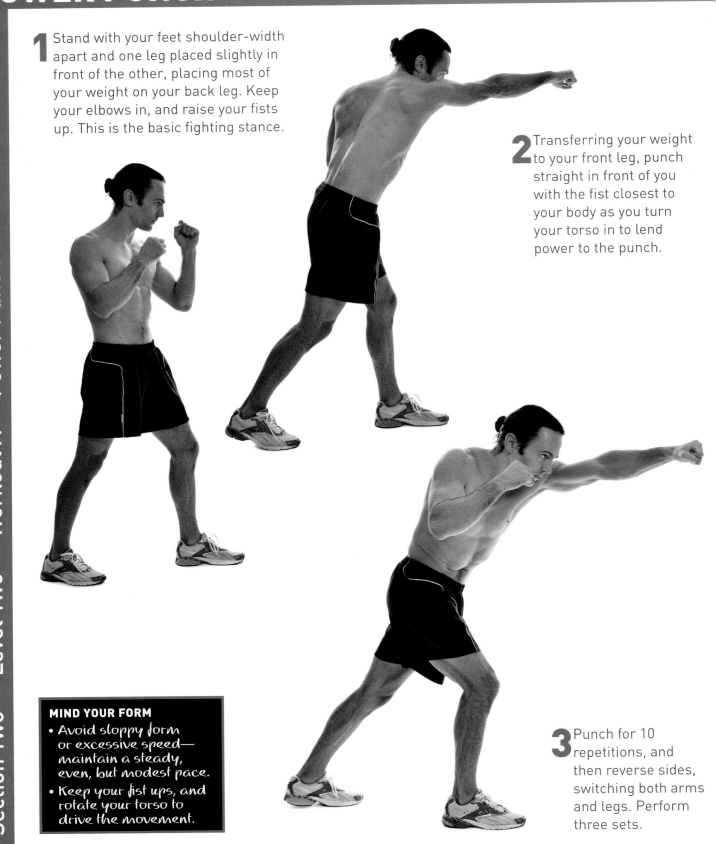

1 Stand with your feet shoulder-width apart and one leg placed slightly in front of the other, placing most of your weight on your back leg. Keep your elbows in, and raise your fists up. This is the basic fighting stance.

2 Transferring your weight to your front leg, punch straight in front of you with the fist closest to your body as you turn your torso in to lend power to the punch.

3 Punch for 10 repetitions, and then reverse sides, switching both arms and legs. Perform three sets.

MIND YOUR FORM
- Avoid sloppy form or excessive speed—maintain a steady, even, but modest pace.
- Keep your fist ups, and rotate your torso to drive the movement.

TYPE
• Cardio

TARGET
• Core
• Arms
• Back

EQUIPMENT
• None

MAJOR TARGETED MUSCLES

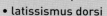

- obliquus internus
- obliquus externus
- rectus abdominis
- serratus anteior
- deltoideus anterior
- deltoideus medialis
- deltoideus posterior
- latissismus dorsi

ANNOTATION KEY

BOLD = MAJOR TARGETED MUSCLES
LIGHT = SECONDARY MUSCLES
* INDICATES DEEP MUSCLES

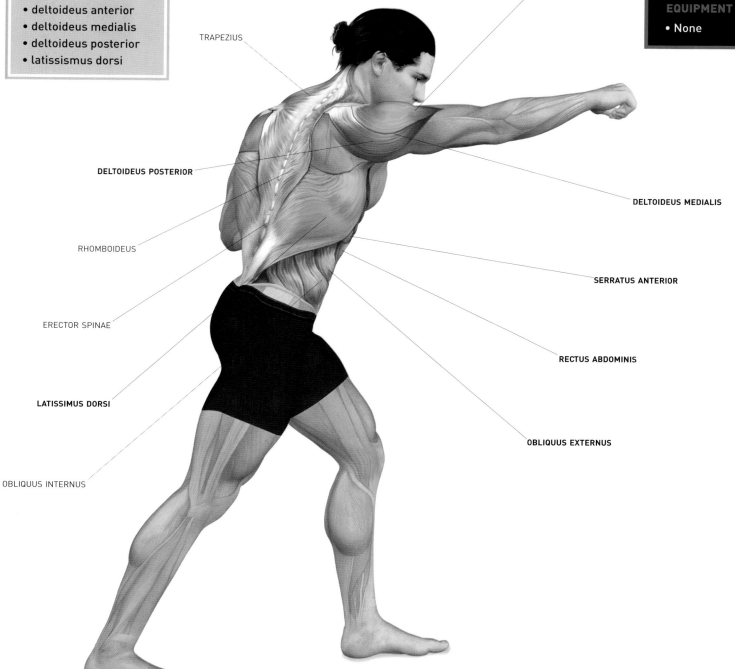

DELTOIDEUS ANTERIOR

TRAPEZIUS

DELTOIDEUS POSTERIOR

DELTOIDEUS MEDIALIS

RHOMBOIDEUS

SERRATUS ANTERIOR

ERECTOR SPINAE

RECTUS ABDOMINIS

LATISSIMUS DORSI

OBLIQUUS EXTERNUS

OBLIQUUS INTERNUS

STAR JUMP

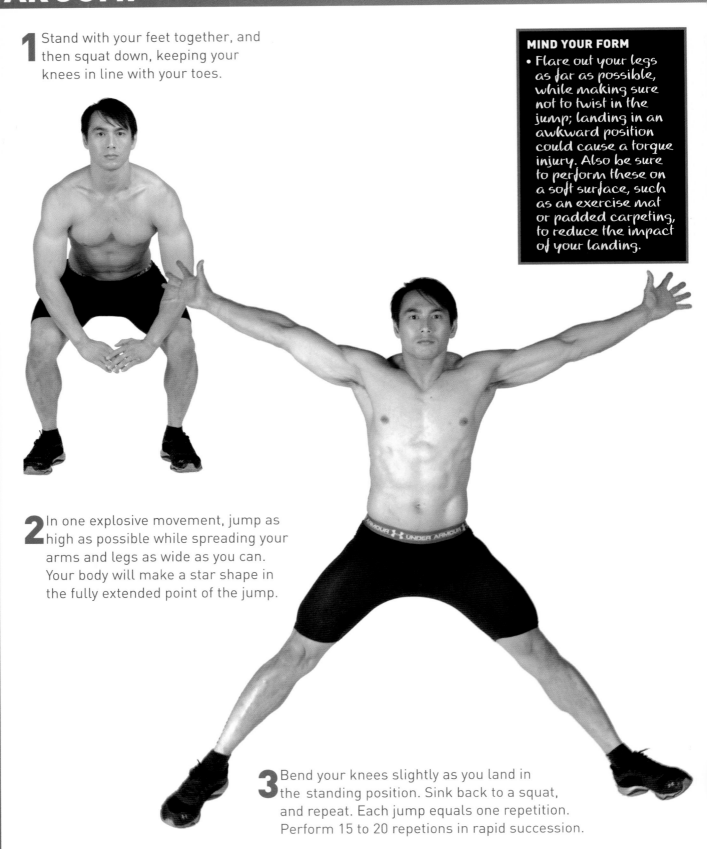

1 Stand with your feet together, and then squat down, keeping your knees in line with your toes.

MIND YOUR FORM
• Flare out your legs as far as possible, while making sure not to twist in the jump; landing in an awkward position could cause a torque injury. Also be sure to perform these on a soft surface, such as an exercise mat or padded carpeting, to reduce the impact of your landing.

2 In one explosive movement, jump as high as possible while spreading your arms and legs as wide as you can. Your body will make a star shape in the fully extended point of the jump.

3 Bend your knees slightly as you land in the standing position. Sink back to a squat, and repeat. Each jump equals one repetition. Perform 15 to 20 repetions in rapid succession.

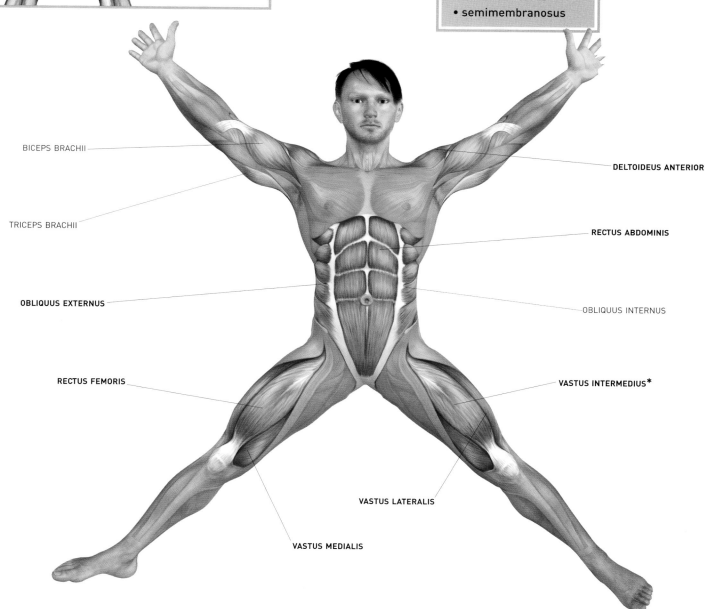

ERECTOR SPINAE

GLUTEUS MAXIMUS

OBTURATOR EXTERNUS

ADDUCTOR MAGNUS

BICEPS FEMORIS

SEMITENDINOSUS

SEMIMEMBRANOSUS

MAJOR TARGETED MUSCLES

- gluteus maximus
- rectus femoris
- vastus medialis
- vastus lateralis
- obliquus externus
- rectus abdominis
- deltoideus anterior
- biceps femoris
- semitendinosus
- semimembranosus

TYPE
- Cardio

TARGET
- Full body

EQUIPMENT
- None

BICEPS BRACHII

TRICEPS BRACHII

OBLIQUUS EXTERNUS

RECTUS FEMORIS

DELTOIDEUS ANTERIOR

RECTUS ABDOMINIS

OBLIQUUS INTERNUS

VASTUS INTERMEDIUS*

VASTUS LATERALIS

VASTUS MEDIALIS

LATERAL BOUNDING

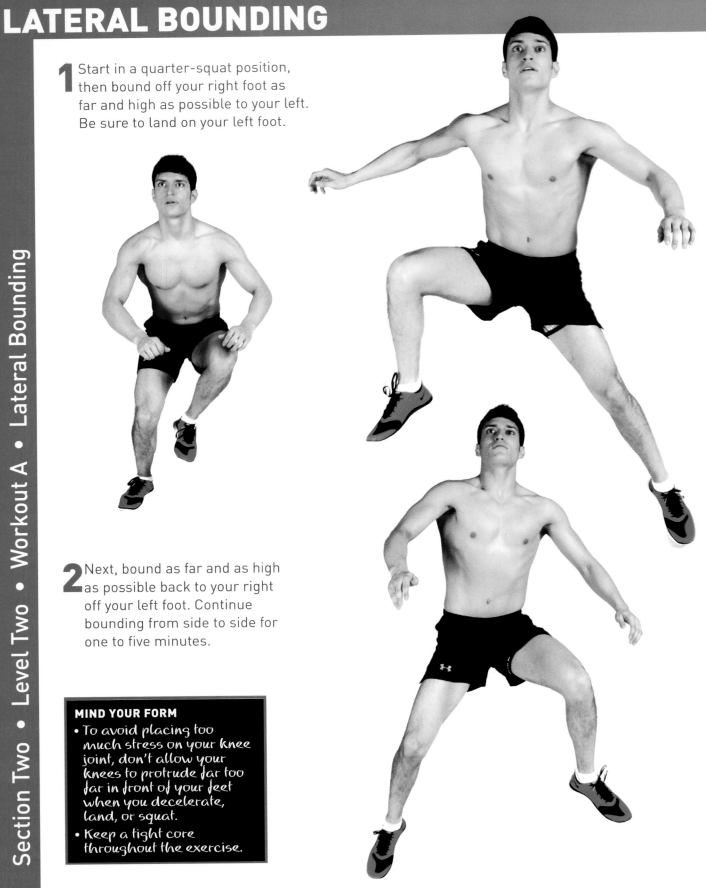

1 Start in a quarter-squat position, then bound off your right foot as far and high as possible to your left. Be sure to land on your left foot.

2 Next, bound as far and as high as possible back to your right off your left foot. Continue bounding from side to side for one to five minutes.

MIND YOUR FORM
- To avoid placing too much stress on your knee joint, don't allow your knees to protrude far too far in front of your feet when you decelerate, land, or squat.
- Keep a tight core throughout the exercise.

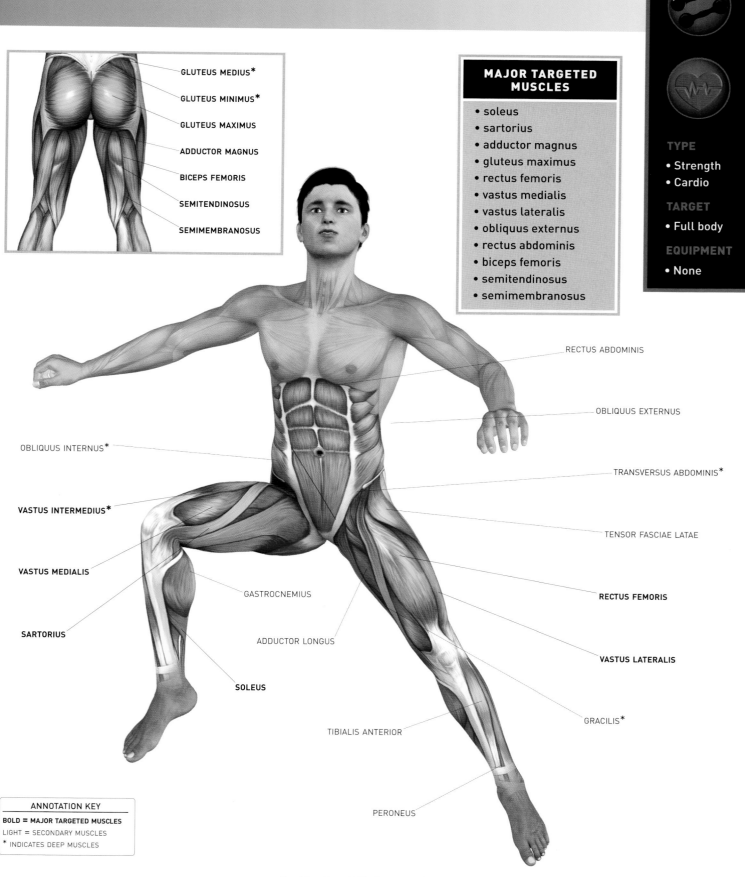

GLUTEUS MEDIUS*

GLUTEUS MINIMUS*

GLUTEUS MAXIMUS

ADDUCTOR MAGNUS

BICEPS FEMORIS

SEMITENDINOSUS

SEMIMEMBRANOSUS

MAJOR TARGETED MUSCLES

- soleus
- sartorius
- adductor magnus
- gluteus maximus
- rectus femoris
- vastus medialis
- vastus lateralis
- obliquus externus
- rectus abdominis
- biceps femoris
- semitendinosus
- semimembranosus

TYPE
- Strength
- Cardio

TARGET
- Full body

EQUIPMENT
- None

RECTUS ABDOMINIS

OBLIQUUS EXTERNUS

OBLIQUUS INTERNUS*

TRANSVERSUS ABDOMINIS*

VASTUS INTERMEDIUS*

TENSOR FASCIAE LATAE

VASTUS MEDIALIS

GASTROCNEMIUS

RECTUS FEMORIS

SARTORIUS

ADDUCTOR LONGUS

VASTUS LATERALIS

SOLEUS

GRACILIS*

TIBIALIS ANTERIOR

PERONEUS

ANNOTATION KEY

BOLD = MAJOR TARGETED MUSCLES

LIGHT = SECONDARY MUSCLES

* INDICATES DEEP MUSCLES

WALKING LUNGE

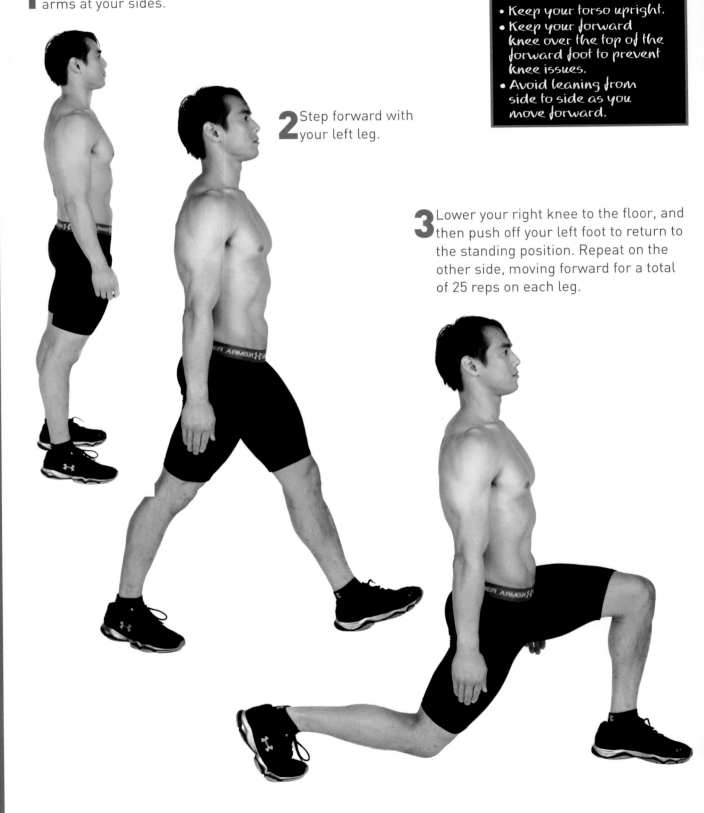

1 Stand tall with your arms at your sides.

2 Step forward with your left leg.

3 Lower your right knee to the floor, and then push off your left foot to return to the standing position. Repeat on the other side, moving forward for a total of 25 reps on each leg.

MIND YOUR FORM
- Keep your torso upright.
- Keep your forward knee over the top of the forward foot to prevent knee issues.
- Avoid leaning from side to side as you move forward.

MAJOR TARGETED MUSCLES

- rectus femoris
- vastus lateralis
- vastus intermedius
- vastus medialis
- soleus
- gastrocnemius
- biceps femoris
- semitendinosus
- semimembranosus
- gluteus maximus

ANNOTATION KEY

BOLD = MAJOR TARGETED MUSCLES
LIGHT = SECONDARY MUSCLES
* INDICATES DEEP MUSCLES

TYPE
- Strength
- Cardio

TARGET
- Lower body

EQUIPMENT
- None

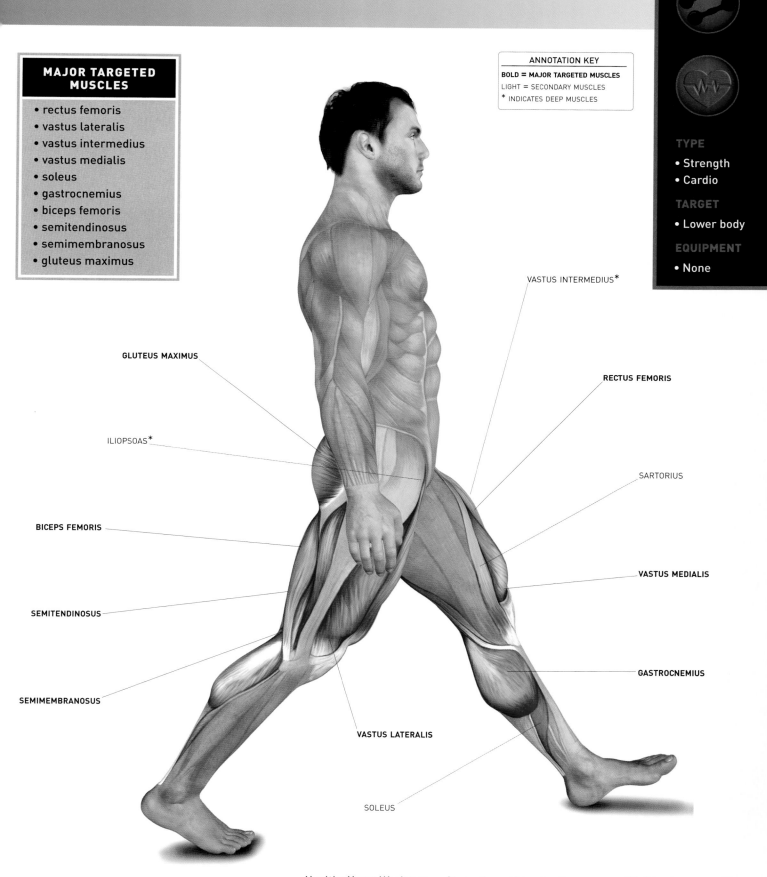

VASTUS INTERMEDIUS*

GLUTEUS MAXIMUS

RECTUS FEMORIS

ILIOPSOAS*

SARTORIUS

BICEPS FEMORIS

VASTUS MEDIALIS

SEMITENDINOSUS

GASTROCNEMIUS

SEMIMEMBRANOSUS

VASTUS LATERALIS

SOLEUS

LEG-EXTENSION CHAIR DIP

1 Sit on the very edge of a chair, with your palms on the seat. Your back should be straight, your knees bent to form 90-degree angles.

2 Slowly and with control, engage your abdominal muscles and press your palms into the seat as you move your buttocks forward and lower slightly so that you are no longer resting on the chair.

3 Bending your arms slightly, extend your left leg forward to form a straight line.

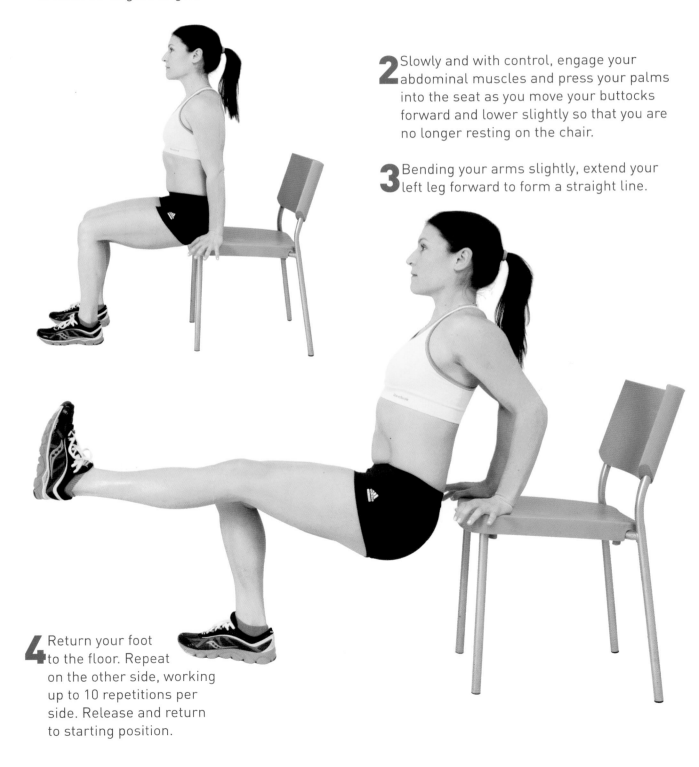

4 Return your foot to the floor. Repeat on the other side, working up to 10 repetitions per side. Release and return to starting position.

MAJOR TARGETED MUSCLES

- coracobrachialis
- deltoideus posterior
- pectoralis minor
- pectoralis major
- biceps brachii
- latissimus dorsi
- rectus abdominis

TYPE
- Strength

TARGET
- Upper body
- Glutes

EQUIPMENT
- Chair

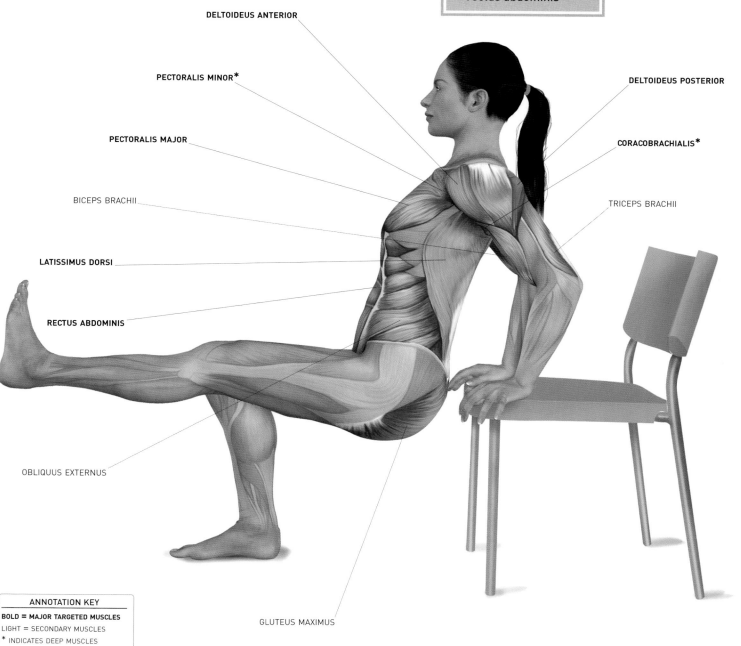

DELTOIDEUS ANTERIOR

PECTORALIS MINOR*

PECTORALIS MAJOR

BICEPS BRACHII

LATISSIMUS DORSI

RECTUS ABDOMINIS

OBLIQUUS EXTERNUS

GLUTEUS MAXIMUS

DELTOIDEUS POSTERIOR

CORACOBRACHIALIS*

TRICEPS BRACHII

ANNOTATION KEY

BOLD = MAJOR TARGETED MUSCLES
LIGHT = SECONDARY MUSCLES
* INDICATES DEEP MUSCLES

SINGLE-LEG CIRCLES

1 Lie faceup flat on a mat, with both legs and arms extended at your sides.

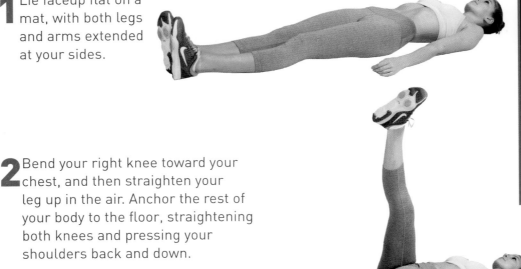

MIND YOUR FORM
- Keep your hips and torso stable while your leg is mobilized.
- Elongate your raised leg from your hip through your foot.
- To maintain stability, avoid making your leg circles too big.

2 Bend your right knee toward your chest, and then straighten your leg up in the air. Anchor the rest of your body to the floor, straightening both knees and pressing your shoulders back and down.

3 Cross your raised leg up and over your body, aiming for your left shoulder. Continue making a circle with the raised leg, returning to the center. Add emphasis to the motion by pausing at the top between repetitions.

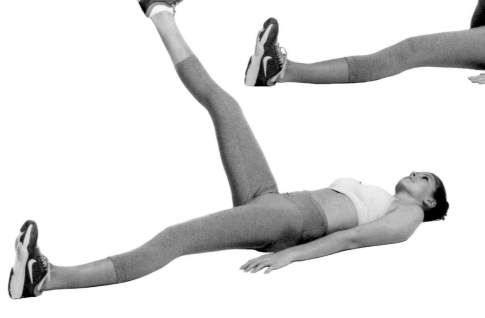

4 Switch directions so that you aim your leg away from your body. Return to the starting position, and then repeat with the other leg. Complete the full movement 10 times with each leg.

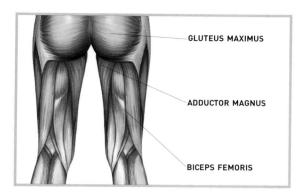

GLUTEUS MAXIMUS

ADDUCTOR MAGNUS

BICEPS FEMORIS

TYPE
• Strength
TARGET
• Abdominals
• Lower body
EQUIPMENT
• Mat

MAJOR TARGETED MUSCLES

• rectus abdominis
• obliquus externus
• rectus femoris
• biceps femoris
• triceps brachii
• gluteus maximus
• adductor magnus
• vastus lateralis
• vastus medialis
• tensor fasciae latae

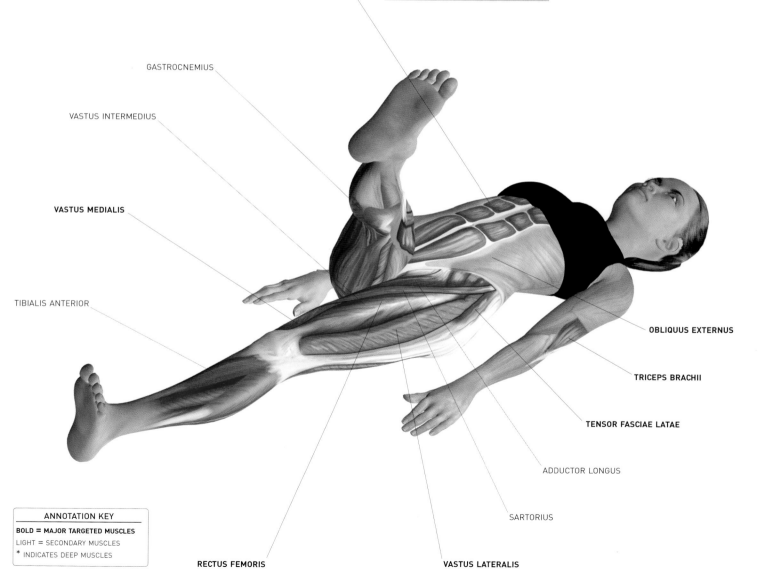

RECTUS ABDOMINIS

GASTROCNEMIUS

VASTUS INTERMEDIUS

VASTUS MEDIALIS

TIBIALIS ANTERIOR

OBLIQUUS EXTERNUS

TRICEPS BRACHII

TENSOR FASCIAE LATAE

ADDUCTOR LONGUS

SARTORIUS

RECTUS FEMORIS

VASTUS LATERALIS

ANNOTATION KEY

BOLD = MAJOR TARGETED MUSCLES
LIGHT = SECONDARY MUSCLES
* INDICATES DEEP MUSCLES

ROLL-UP TRICEPS LIFT

1 Lie on the floor, with your spine in a neutral position. Hold a body bar in both hands. Bend your elbows so that your arms form a right angle with the body bar above your head.

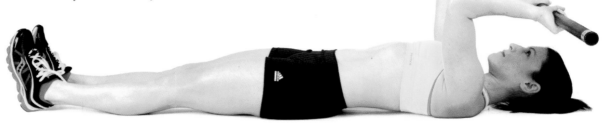

2 Keeping the rest of your body in place, straighten your arms.

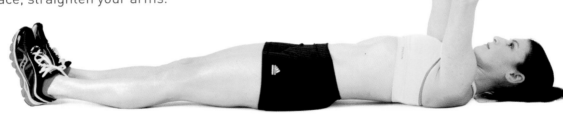

MIND YOUR FORM
- Keep the rest of your body stable as you move smoothly and with control.
- Strongly engage your abdominal muscles as you roll up and down.
- Avoid Moving in a jerky manner.

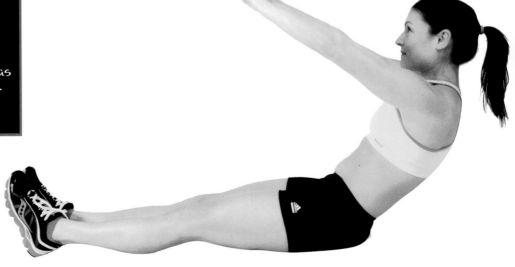

3 Maintaining this arm position, use your core muscles to smoothly roll up to a sitting position. Keep your arms extended, with the body bar lifted overhead.

4 Slowly roll back to lie in the starting position. Repeat, completing 10 repetitions.

TYPE
• Strength

TARGET
• Core
• Upper arms

EQUIPMENT
• Barbell

MAJOR TARGETED MUSCLES

• triceps brachii
• rectus abdominis
• transversus abdominis*
• erector spinae*
• obliquus externus

ANNOTATION KEY

BOLD = MAJOR TARGETED MUSCLES
LIGHT = SECONDARY MUSCLES
* INDICATES DEEP MUSCLES

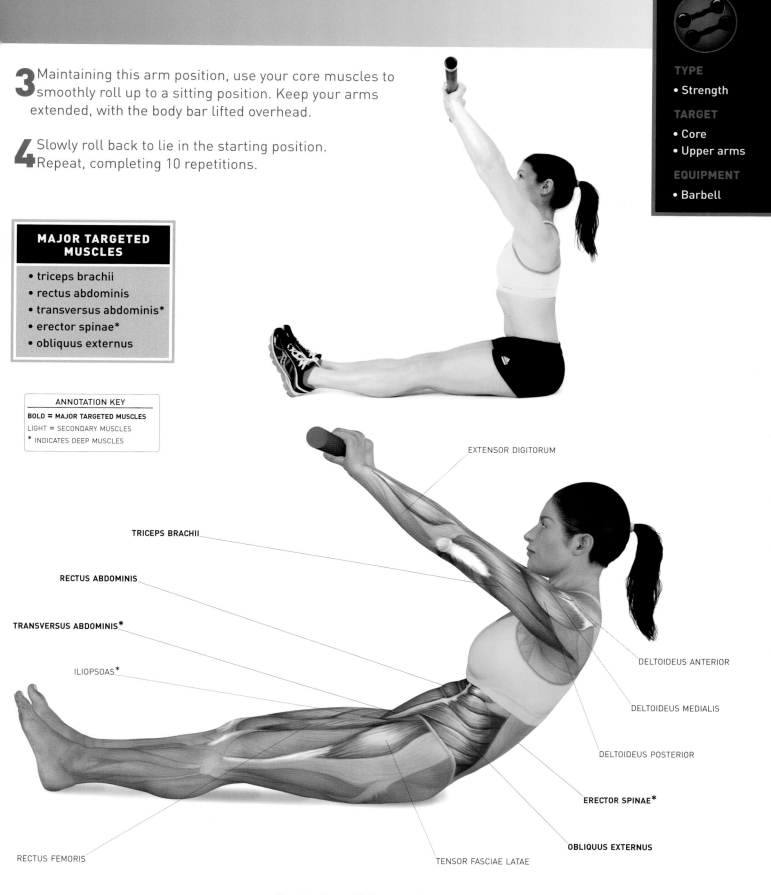

EXTENSOR DIGITORUM

TRICEPS BRACHII

RECTUS ABDOMINIS

TRANSVERSUS ABDOMINIS*

ILIOPSOAS*

DELTOIDEUS ANTERIOR

DELTOIDEUS MEDIALIS

DELTOIDEUS POSTERIOR

ERECTOR SPINAE*

OBLIQUUS EXTERNUS

RECTUS FEMORIS

TENSOR FASCIAE LATAE

SEATED RUSSIAN TWIST

1 Holding a dumbbell in both hands, sit with your legs extended in front of you, knees bent and feet about hip-width apart. Lean back slightly.

MIND YOUR FORM
- Anchor your heels to the floor.
- Avoid swinging your arms or moving in a jerky manner.
- Avoid arching or rounding your back

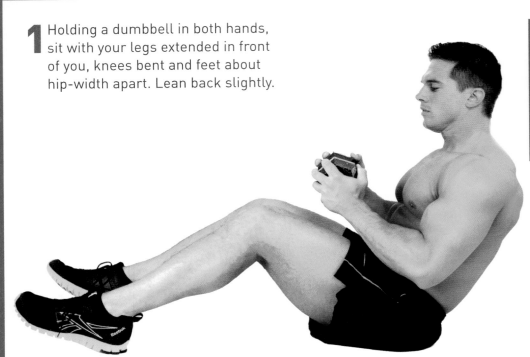

2 Engage your core muscles as you bring the dumbbell to the right side.

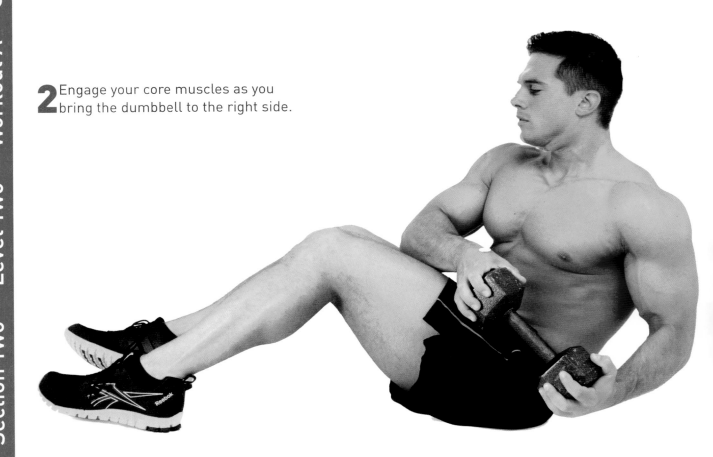

3 Bring the dumbbell to the middle of your body and then to the left side. Continue to alternate for a total of 20 repetitions on each side.

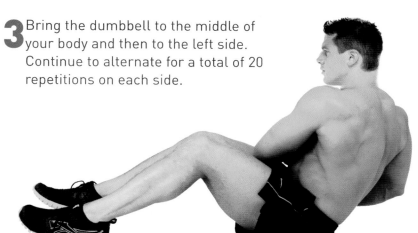

MAJOR TARGETED MUSCLES

- obliquus internus
- obliquus externus
- rectus abdominis
- latissimus dorsi
- biceps brachii
- triceps brachii
- rectus femoris
- iliopsoas

TYPE
- Strength

TARGET
- Core
- Upper arms

EQUIPMENT
- Dumbbells

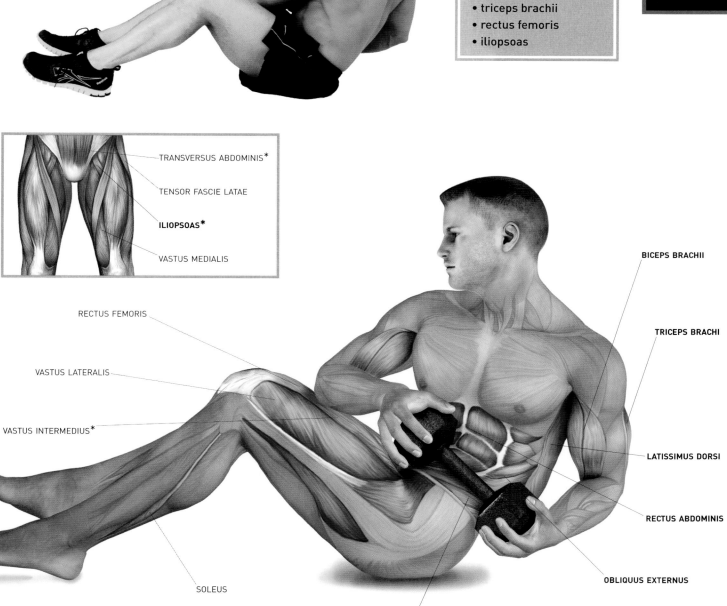

TRANSVERSUS ABDOMINIS*

TENSOR FASCIE LATAE

ILIOPSOAS*

VASTUS MEDIALIS

RECTUS FEMORIS

VASTUS LATERALIS

VASTUS INTERMEDIUS*

SOLEUS

BICEPS BRACHII

TRICEPS BRACHI

LATISSIMUS DORSI

RECTUS ABDOMINIS

OBLIQUUS EXTERNUS

OBLIQUUS INTERNUS

ANNOTATION KEY

BOLD = MAJOR TARGETED MUSCLES
LIGHT = SECONDARY MUSCLES
* INDICATES DEEP MUSCLES

BEAR CRAWL

1 Place both hands and feet on the floor.

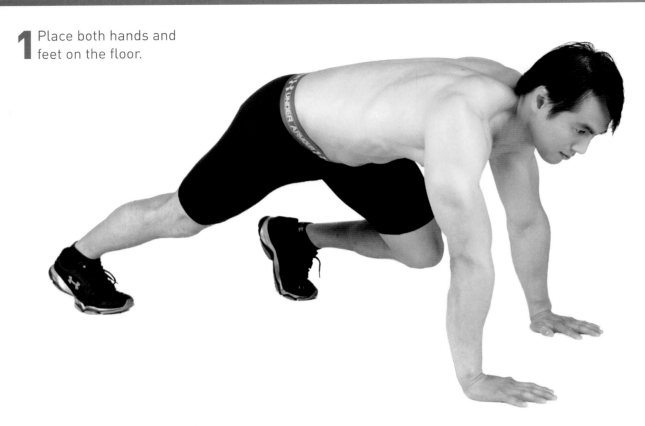

2 Walk your left arm and right leg forward, and then your right arm and left leg.

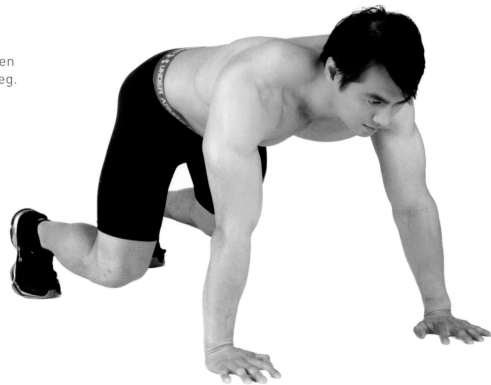

MIND YOUR FORM
- Move as steadily and as smoothly as possible, being careful to distribute your weight and not placing all of your weight on your arms and shoulders, which can stress your rotator cuffs.
- Avoid touching your knees to the floor.

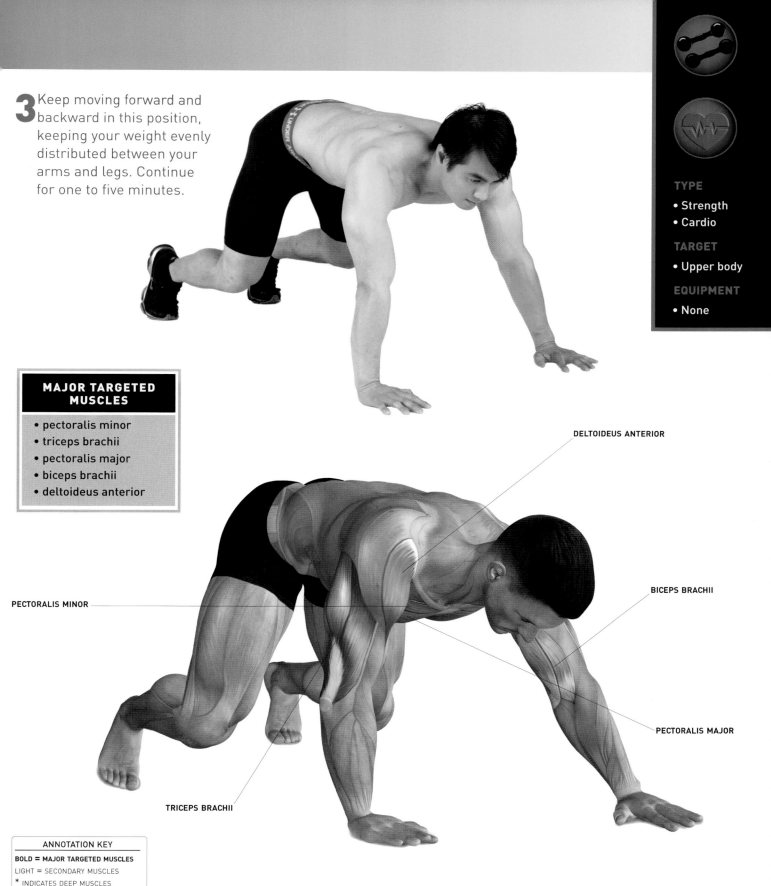

3 Keep moving forward and backward in this position, keeping your weight evenly distributed between your arms and legs. Continue for one to five minutes.

TYPE
• Strength
• Cardio

TARGET
• Upper body

EQUIPMENT
• None

MAJOR TARGETED MUSCLES

• pectoralis minor
• triceps brachii
• pectoralis major
• biceps brachii
• deltoideus anterior

DELTOIDEUS ANTERIOR

BICEPS BRACHII

PECTORALIS MINOR

PECTORALIS MAJOR

TRICEPS BRACHII

ANNOTATION KEY

BOLD = MAJOR TARGETED MUSCLES
LIGHT = SECONDARY MUSCLES
* INDICATES DEEP MUSCLES

CROSSOVER STEP-UP

1 Stand with your feet hip-width apart, holding a medicine ball in front of your chest. Position a high step and a lower step beside your left foot.

2 Cross your right leg over your left, resting it on the step. Shift weight onto your right foot to step up.

MIND YOUR FORM
- Keep holding the medicine ball in front of your chest.
- Maintain a steady pace.
- Keep your torso facing forward.
- Pull your abdominal muscles inward to keep them engaged.
- Gaze forward.
- Press your shoulders away from your ears.
- Avoid twisting your neck.
- Avoid hunching your shoulders.
- Avoid arching your back or hunching forward.
- Don't move so quickly that you sacrifice form.

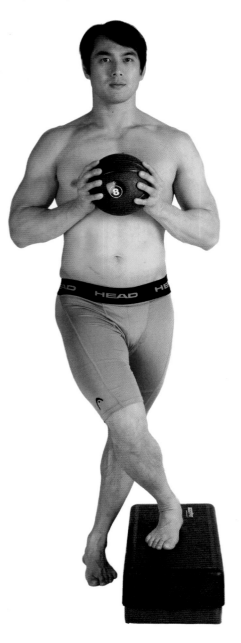

3 Rest your left foot on the lower step.

4 Again cross your right leg over your left to step down onto the floor.

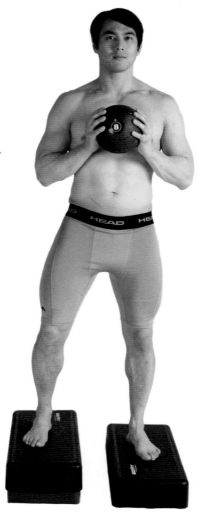

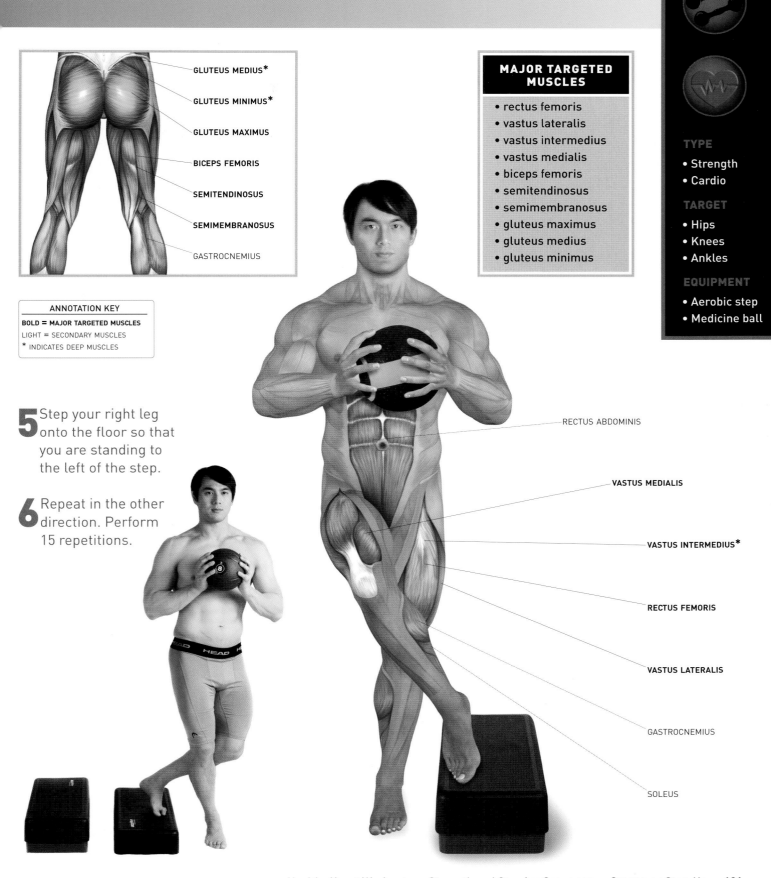

GLUTEUS MEDIUS*

GLUTEUS MINIMUS*

GLUTEUS MAXIMUS

BICEPS FEMORIS

SEMITENDINOSUS

SEMIMEMBRANOSUS

GASTROCNEMIUS

ANNOTATION KEY

BOLD = MAJOR TARGETED MUSCLES

LIGHT = SECONDARY MUSCLES

* INDICATES DEEP MUSCLES

MAJOR TARGETED MUSCLES

- rectus femoris
- vastus lateralis
- vastus intermedius
- vastus medialis
- biceps femoris
- semitendinosus
- semimembranosus
- gluteus maximus
- gluteus medius
- gluteus minimus

TYPE
- Strength
- Cardio

TARGET
- Hips
- Knees
- Ankles

EQUIPMENT
- Aerobic step
- Medicine ball

5 Step your right leg onto the floor so that you are standing to the left of the step.

6 Repeat in the other direction. Perform 15 repetitions.

RECTUS ABDOMINIS

VASTUS MEDIALIS

VASTUS INTERMEDIUS*

RECTUS FEMORIS

VASTUS LATERALIS

GASTROCNEMIUS

SOLEUS

POWER SQUAT

1 Stand with your feet together, holding a weighted medicine ball in front of your torso.

2 Shift your weight to your left foot, and bend your right knee, lifting your right foot toward your buttocks. Bend your elbows, and draw the ball toward the outside of your right ear.

MIND YOUR FORM
- Move the ball in an arc through the air.
- Keep your hips and knees aligned throughout the movement.
- Keep your neck and shoulders relaxed.
- Don't extend your knee beyond your toes as you bend and rotate.
- Keep your foot in the its starting position throughout the exercise.

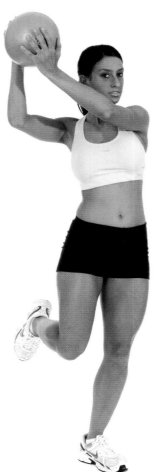

3 Maintaining a neutral spine, bend at your hips and knee. Lower your torso toward your left side, bringing the ball toward your left ankle.

4 Press into your left leg, and straighten your knee and torso, returning to the starting position. Repeat 15 times for two sets on each leg.

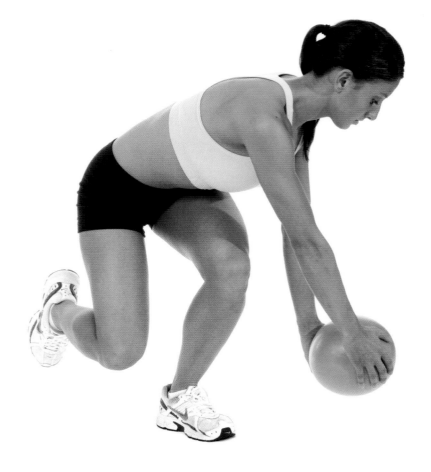

MAJOR TARGETED MUSCLES

- semitendinosus
- semimembranosus
- biceps femoris
- vastus medialis
- vastus lateralis
- rectus femoris
- gluteus maximus
- gluteus medius
- piriformis
- erector spinae
- tibialis anterior
- tibialis posterior
- soleus
- gastrocnemius
- deltoideus medialis
- infraspinatus
- supraspinatus
- teres minor

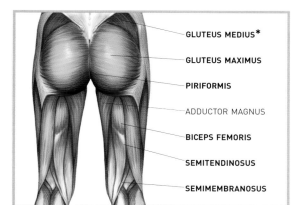

GLUTEUS MEDIUS*
GLUTEUS MAXIMUS
PIRIFORMIS
ADDUCTOR MAGNUS
BICEPS FEMORIS
SEMITENDINOSUS
SEMIMEMBRANOSUS

ANNOTATION KEY

BOLD = MAJOR TARGETED MUSCLES
LIGHT = SECONDARY MUSCLES
* INDICATES DEEP MUSCLES

TYPE
- Strength

TARGET
- Full body

EQUIPMENT
- Medicine ball

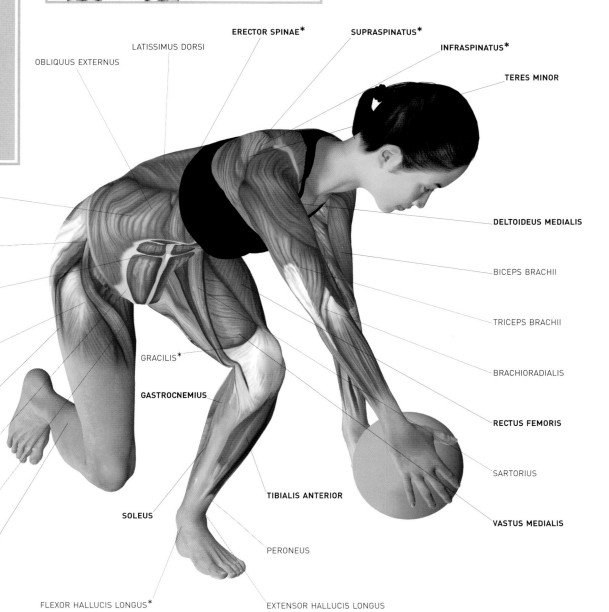

ERECTOR SPINAE*
SUPRASPINATUS*
INFRASPINATUS*
TERES MINOR
LATISSIMUS DORSI
OBLIQUUS EXTERNUS
DELTOIDEUS MEDIALIS
OBLIQUUS INTERNUS*
BICEPS BRACHII
TENSOR FASCIAE LATAE
TRICEPS BRACHII
RECTUS ABDOMINIS
BRACHIORADIALIS
VASTUS INTERMEDIUS*
GRACILIS*
RECTUS FEMORIS
GASTROCNEMIUS
VASTUS LATERALIS
SARTORIUS
TRANSVERSUS ABDOMINIS*
TIBIALIS ANTERIOR
ADDUCTOR LONGUS
VASTUS MEDIALIS
SOLEUS
TIBIALIS POSTERIOR*
PERONEUS
FLEXOR HALLUCIS LONGUS*
EXTENSOR HALLUCIS LONGUS

HIP-TO THIGH STRETCH

1 Kneeling on your right knee, place your left foot in front of you. Your left foot should be flat on the floor, your right heel lifted.

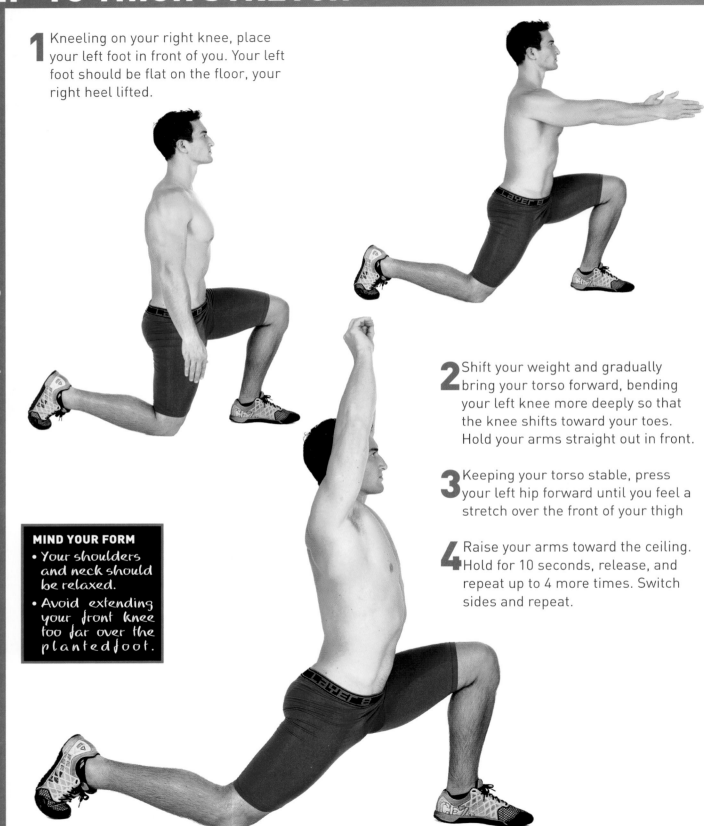

2 Shift your weight and gradually bring your torso forward, bending your left knee more deeply so that the knee shifts toward your toes. Hold your arms straight out in front.

3 Keeping your torso stable, press your left hip forward until you feel a stretch over the front of your thigh

4 Raise your arms toward the ceiling. Hold for 10 seconds, release, and repeat up to 4 more times. Switch sides and repeat.

MIND YOUR FORM
- Your shoulders and neck should be relaxed.
- Avoid extending your front knee too far over the planted foot.

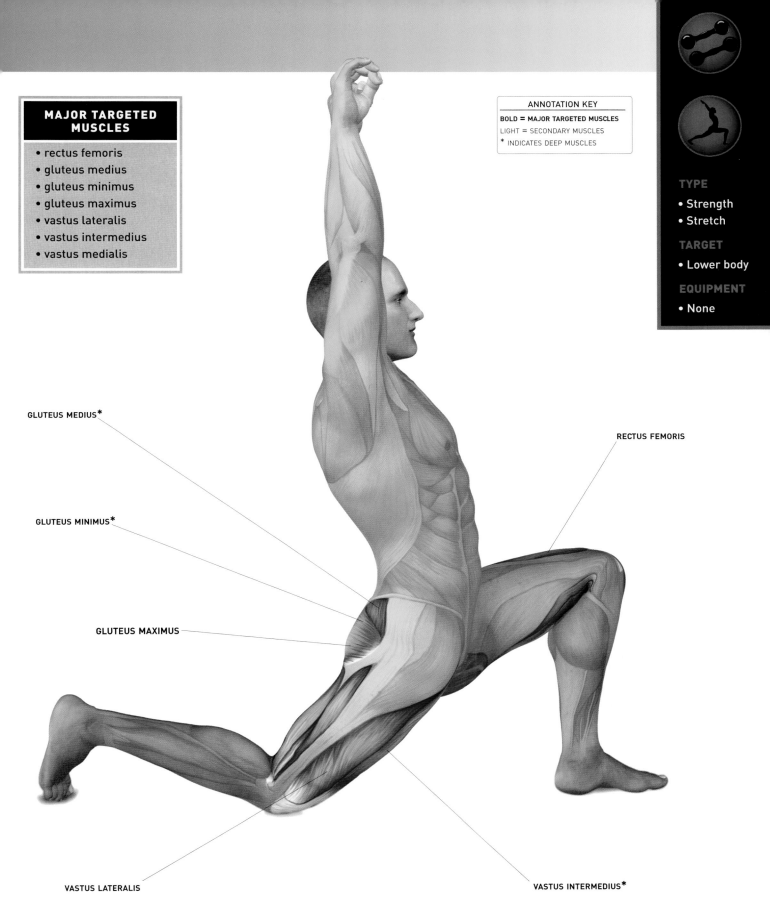

MAJOR TARGETED MUSCLES

- rectus femoris
- gluteus medius
- gluteus minimus
- gluteus maximus
- vastus lateralis
- vastus intermedius
- vastus medialis

ANNOTATION KEY

BOLD = MAJOR TARGETED MUSCLES
LIGHT = SECONDARY MUSCLES
* INDICATES DEEP MUSCLES

TYPE
- Strength
- Stretch

TARGET
- Lower body

EQUIPMENT
- None

GLUTEUS MEDIUS*

GLUTEUS MINIMUS*

GLUTEUS MAXIMUS

VASTUS LATERALIS

RECTUS FEMORIS

VASTUS INTERMEDIUS*

WORKOUT B

Core and Balance Sequence

Start your joint health regimen at the top, with a workout that targets your neck and shoulders. Whether you spend hours at your desk peering at a computer screen or toss heavy weights like a book-laden backpack across your shoulders every day, this area can too often hold a lot of tension. Try this beginner-level workout to help counteract that tightness and keep your shoulder and neck joints moving smoothly.

1. TURKISH GET-UP
(Pages 108–109)

Perform 10 repetitions on each side.

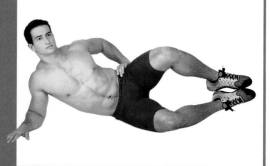

2. FRONT PLANK WITH LEG LIFT
(Pages 110–111)

Perform 10 repetitions on each side.

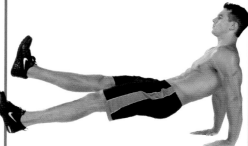

3. BICYCLE CRUNCH
(Pages 112–113)

Alternate sides for 20 repetitions on each side.

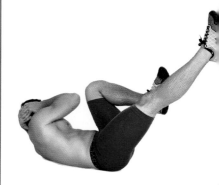

4. CLAMSHELL SERIES
(Pages 114–115)

Perform 10 repetitions on each side.

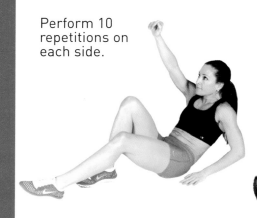

5. TOWEL FLY
(Pages 116–117)

Perform 10 repetitions.

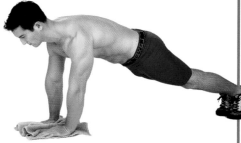

6. BURPEE
(Pages 117–119)

Perform two 60-second sets.

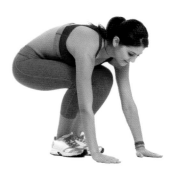

7. MOUNTAIN CLIMBER
(Pages 120–121)

Perform 10 repetitions.

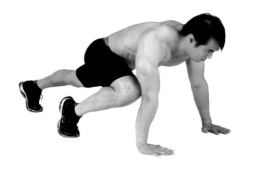

8. REVERSE LUNGE
(Pages 122–123)

Perform two sets of 10 repetitions on each side.

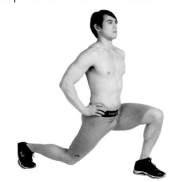

EQUIPMENT CHECKLIST

- ✗ Swiss ball
- ✗ medicine ball
- ✗ dumbbells
- ✗ barbell
- ✔ kettlebells
- ✔ mat
- ✔ chair
- ✔ bench
- ✔ aerobic step
- ✗ towel

9. STEP-UP
(Pages 124–125)

Perform 10 to 12 repetitions on each side.

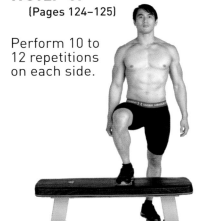

10. INVERTED LEG EXTENSION
(Pages 126–127)

Alternate sides for 10 repetitions on each side.

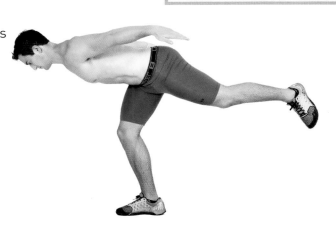

11. LATERAL STEP-OVER
(Pages 128–129)

Perform for two minutes.

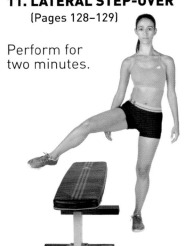

12. SIDE KICK
(Pages 130–131)

Perform two sets, alternating sides for 10 repetitions on each side.

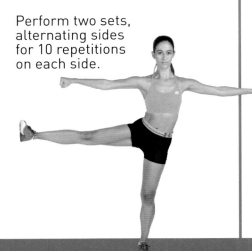

13. SIDE-BEND PLANK
(Pages 132–133)

Perform two times on each side.

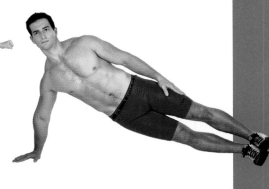

TURKISH GET-UP

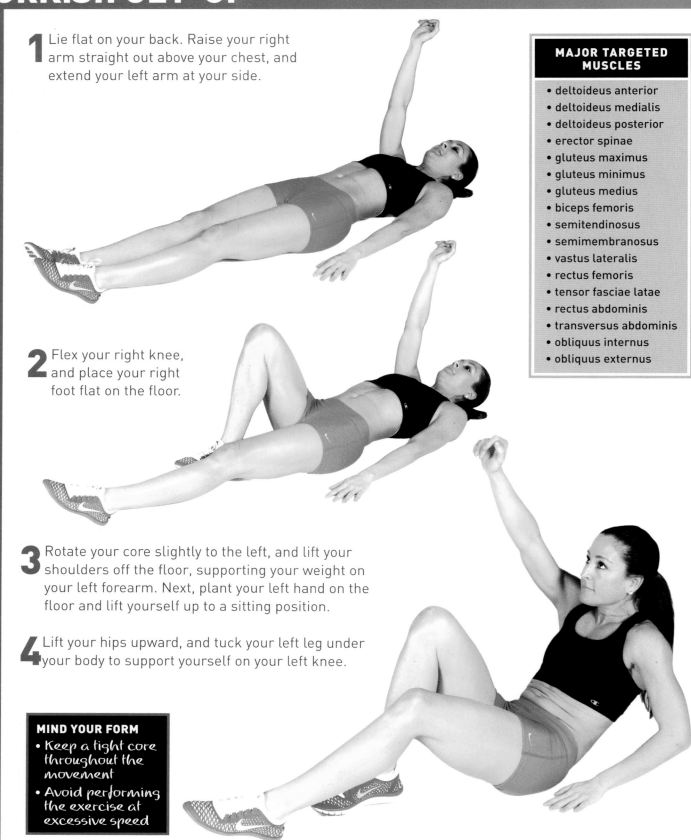

1 Lie flat on your back. Raise your right arm straight out above your chest, and extend your left arm at your side.

MAJOR TARGETED MUSCLES

- deltoideus anterior
- deltoideus medialis
- deltoideus posterior
- erector spinae
- gluteus maximus
- gluteus minimus
- gluteus medius
- biceps femoris
- semitendinosus
- semimembranosus
- vastus lateralis
- rectus femoris
- tensor fasciae latae
- rectus abdominis
- transversus abdominis
- obliquus internus
- obliquus externus

2 Flex your right knee, and place your right foot flat on the floor.

3 Rotate your core slightly to the left, and lift your shoulders off the floor, supporting your weight on your left forearm. Next, plant your left hand on the floor and lift yourself up to a sitting position.

4 Lift your hips upward, and tuck your left leg under your body to support yourself on your left knee.

MIND YOUR FORM
- Keep a tight core throughout the movement
- Avoid performing the exercise at excessive speed

5 Lift your left hand off the floor and push through your right foot to a standing position, keeping your right arm stretched over your head throughout the exercise.

6 Return to the starting position. Perform 10 repetitions per arm.

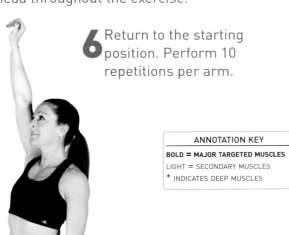

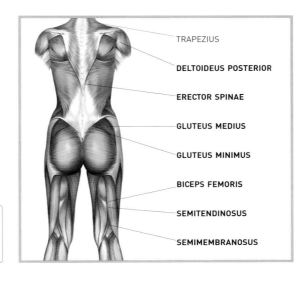

TRAPEZIUS

DELTOIDEUS POSTERIOR

ERECTOR SPINAE

GLUTEUS MEDIUS

GLUTEUS MINIMUS

BICEPS FEMORIS

SEMITENDINOSUS

SEMIMEMBRANOSUS

ANNOTATION KEY
BOLD = MAJOR TARGETED MUSCLES
LIGHT = SECONDARY MUSCLES
* INDICATES DEEP MUSCLES

TYPE
• Strength

TARGET
• Full body

EQUIPMENT
• Mat

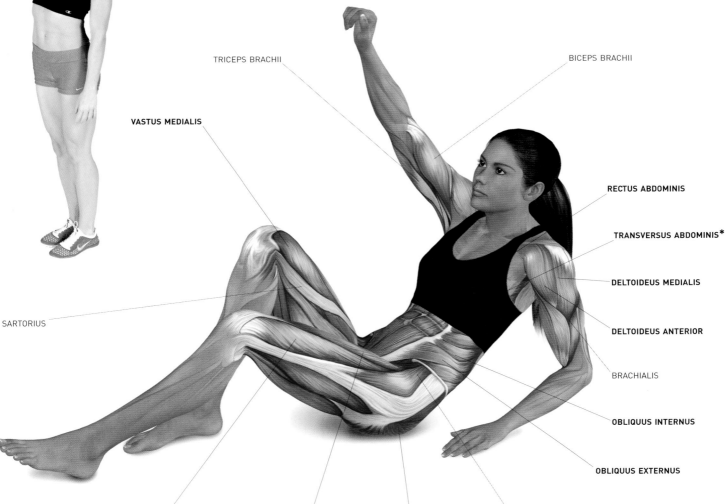

TRICEPS BRACHII

BICEPS BRACHII

VASTUS MEDIALIS

RECTUS ABDOMINIS

TRANSVERSUS ABDOMINIS*

SARTORIUS

DELTOIDEUS MEDIALIS

DELTOIDEUS ANTERIOR

BRACHIALIS

OBLIQUUS INTERNUS

OBLIQUUS EXTERNUS

VASTUS LATERALIS

RECTUS FEMORIS

GLUTEUS MAXIMUS

TENSOR FASCIAE LATAE

FRONT PLANK WITH LEG LIFT

1 Sit with your legs extended in front of you and your arms directly behind you, with your fingers pointing straight ahead.

2 Push through your palms and raise your hips and glutes off the ground until your body forms a straight line from the shoulders.

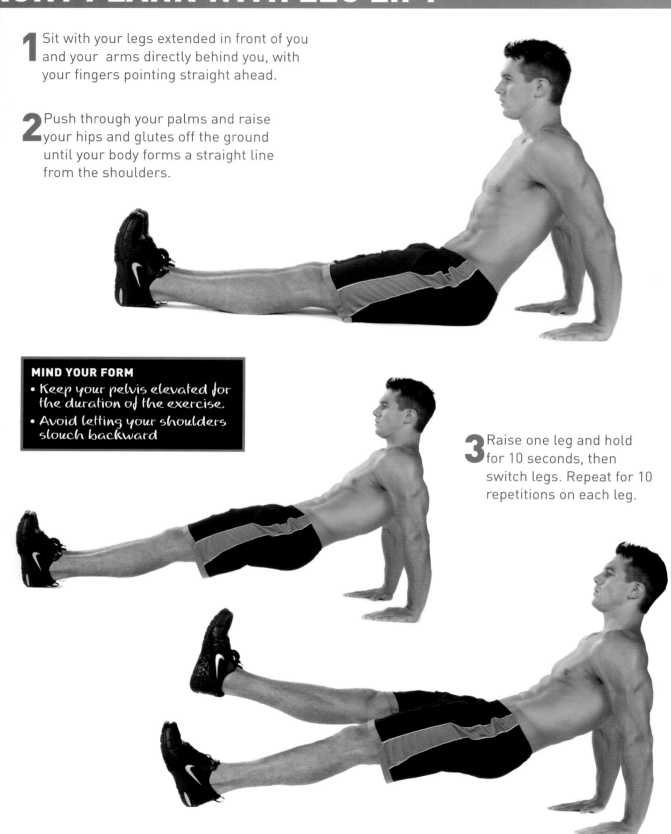

MIND YOUR FORM
- Keep your pelvis elevated for the duration of the exercise.
- Avoid letting your shoulders slouch backward

3 Raise one leg and hold for 10 seconds, then switch legs. Repeat for 10 repetitions on each leg.

MAJOR TARGETED MUSCLES

- latissimus dorsi
- obliquus externus
- obliquus internus
- rectus abdominis
- transversus abdominis
- tensor fasciae latae
- transversus abdominis
- rectus femoris
- gluteus medius
- gluteus maximus

ANNOTATION KEY

BOLD = MAJOR TARGETED MUSCLES
LIGHT = SECONDARY MUSCLES
* INDICATES DEEP MUSCLES

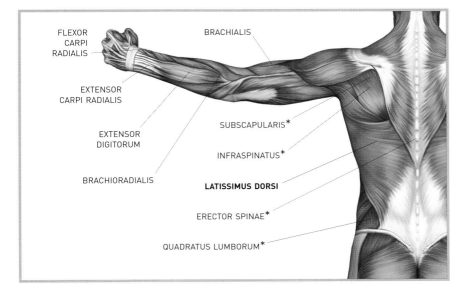

FLEXOR CARPI RADIALIS
BRACHIALIS
EXTENSOR CARPI RADIALIS
EXTENSOR DIGITORUM
BRACHIORADIALIS
SUBSCAPULARIS*
INFRASPINATUS*
LATISSIMUS DORSI
ERECTOR SPINAE*
QUADRATUS LUMBORUM*

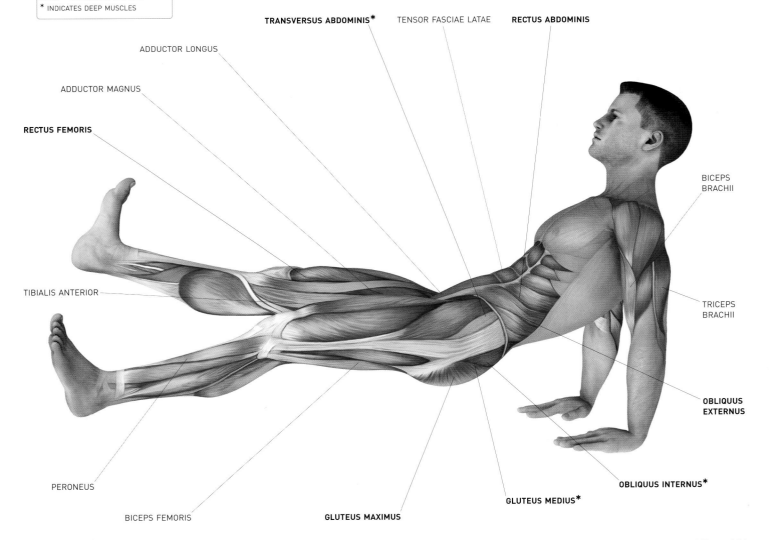

TRANSVERSUS ABDOMINIS*
TENSOR FASCIAE LATAE
RECTUS ABDOMINIS
ADDUCTOR LONGUS
ADDUCTOR MAGNUS
RECTUS FEMORIS
BICEPS BRACHII
TIBIALIS ANTERIOR
TRICEPS BRACHII
OBLIQUUS EXTERNUS
PERONEUS
OBLIQUUS INTERNUS*
BICEPS FEMORIS
GLUTEUS MAXIMUS
GLUTEUS MEDIUS*

BICYCLE CRUNCH

1 Lie supine on the floor with your knees bent. Bring your hands behind your head, lifting your legs off the floor

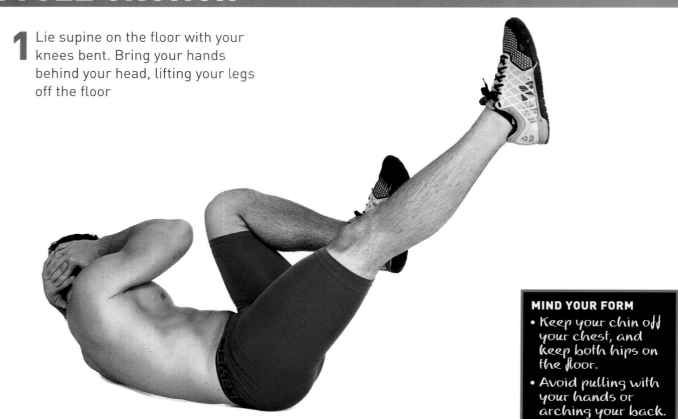

MIND YOUR FORM
- Keep your chin off your chest, and keep both hips on the floor.
- Avoid pulling with your hands or arching your back.

2 Roll up with your torso, reaching your left elbow to your right knee while extending the left leg in front of you. Imagine pulling your shoulder blades off the floor and twisting from your ribs and oblique muscles.

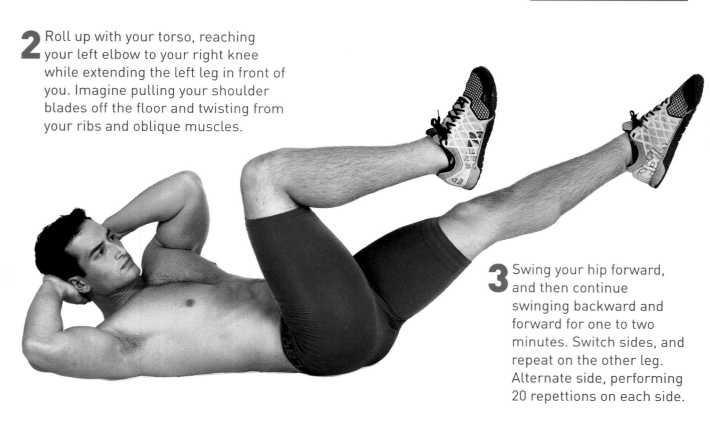

3 Swing your hip forward, and then continue swinging backward and forward for one to two minutes. Switch sides, and repeat on the other leg. Alternate side, performing 20 repettions on each side.

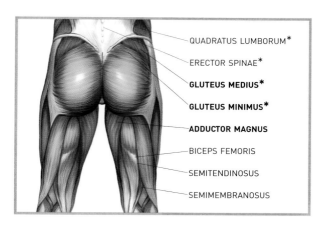

QUADRATUS LUMBORUM*
ERECTOR SPINAE*
GLUTEUS MEDIUS*
GLUTEUS MINIMUS*
ADDUCTOR MAGNUS
BICEPS FEMORIS
SEMITENDINOSUS
SEMIMEMBRANOSUS

ANNOTATION KEY

BOLD = MAJOR TARGETED MUSCLES
LIGHT = SECONDARY MUSCLES
* INDICATES DEEP MUSCLES

MAJOR TARGETED MUSCLES

- rectus abdominis
- triceps brachii
- biceps brachii
- deltoideus anterior
- adductor magnus
- gluteus medius*
- gluteus minimus*
- gluteus maximus
- tensor fasciae latae
- obliquus externus
- obliquus internus

TYPE
- Strength
- Cardio

TARGET
- Abdominals
- Lower body
- Upper arms

EQUIPMENT
- None

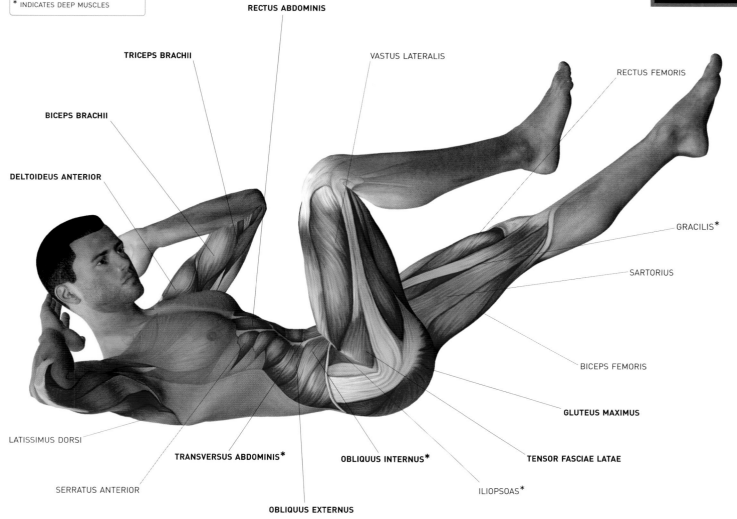

RECTUS ABDOMINIS
TRICEPS BRACHII
VASTUS LATERALIS
RECTUS FEMORIS
BICEPS BRACHII
DELTOIDEUS ANTERIOR
GRACILIS*
SARTORIUS
BICEPS FEMORIS
LATISSIMUS DORSI
GLUTEUS MAXIMUS
TRANSVERSUS ABDOMINIS*
OBLIQUUS INTERNUS*
TENSOR FASCIAE LATAE
SERRATUS ANTERIOR
ILIOPSOAS*
OBLIQUUS EXTERNUS

CLAMSHELL SERIES

1 Lie on your right side on a mat with your knees bent and stacked on top of each other. Bend your left elbow, placing it directly underneath your shoulder so that your forearm is supporting your upper body. Place your left hand on your hip.

MIND YOUR FORM
- Keep your hips stacked and pulled forward slightly.
- Press your shoulder and forearm into the floor throughout the exercise.
- Relax your neck and shoulders.
- Avoid allowing your hips to move while your lift your knee.

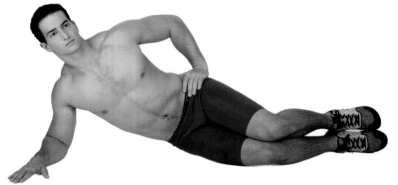

2 Without moving your hips, open your left knee upward, and then return to the starting position. Repeat 10 times.

3 Lift both ankles off the floor, making sure to maintain a straight line with your torso.

4 While your ankles are still lifted, lift and lower your left knee to open and close your legs. Repeat 10 times.

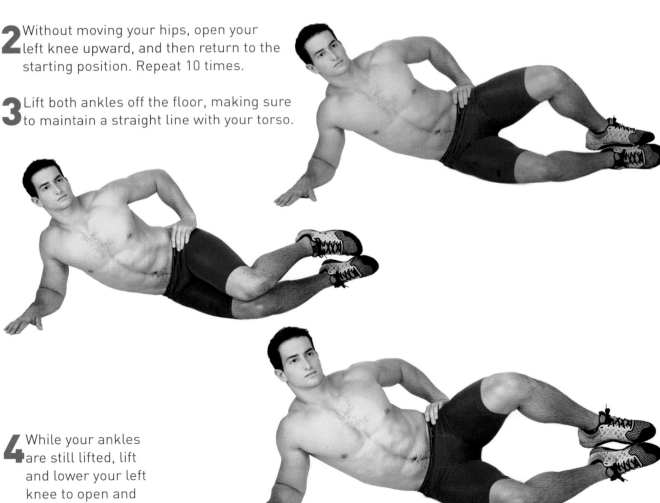

Section Two • Level Two • Workout B • Clamshell Series

114

5 The final part of this series begins with both ankles elevated. Lift your left knee to separate your legs, and then straighten your left leg, being careful not to move the position of your thigh. Bend your knee, and return to the starting position. Repeat 10 times, switch sides, and start from the beginning.

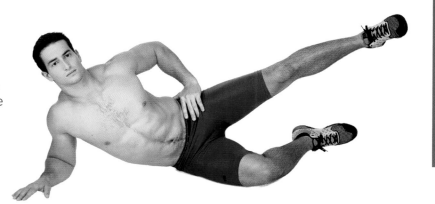

TYPE
- Strength

TARGET
- Abdominals
- Lower body
- Upper arms

EQUIPMENT
- Mat

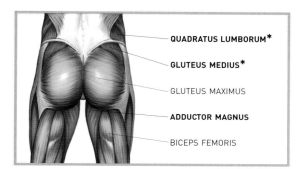

QUADRATUS LUMBORUM*

GLUTEUS MEDIUS*

GLUTEUS MAXIMUS

ADDUCTOR MAGNUS

BICEPS FEMORIS

ANNOTATION KEY
BOLD = MAJOR TARGETED MUSCLES
LIGHT = SECONDARY MUSCLES
* INDICATES DEEP MUSCLES

MAJOR TARGETED MUSCLES

- rectus abdominis
- obliquus internus
- obliquus externus
- tensor fasciae latae
- adductor magnus
- adductor longus
- iliopsoas
- gluteus medius
- quadratus lumborum

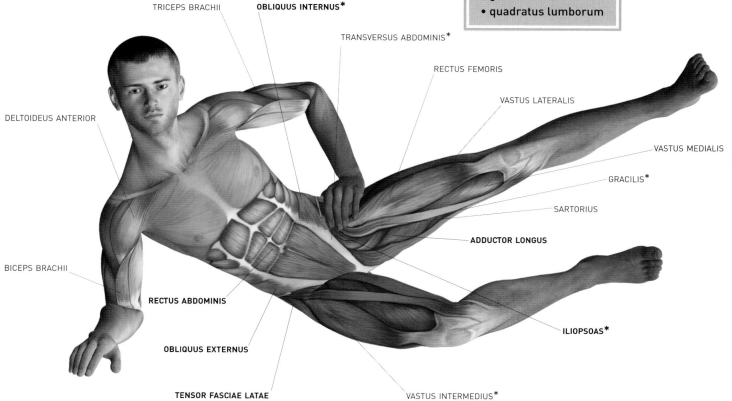

TRICEPS BRACHII

OBLIQUUS INTERNUS*

TRANSVERSUS ABDOMINIS*

RECTUS FEMORIS

VASTUS LATERALIS

DELTOIDEUS ANTERIOR

VASTUS MEDIALIS

GRACILIS*

SARTORIUS

ADDUCTOR LONGUS

BICEPS BRACHII

ILIOPSOAS*

RECTUS ABDOMINIS

OBLIQUUS EXTERNUS

TENSOR FASCIAE LATAE

VASTUS INTERMEDIUS*

TOWEL FLY

1 Place a towel on the floor in front of you. Assume the push-up position, with your elbows fully extended, and the towel under your hands.

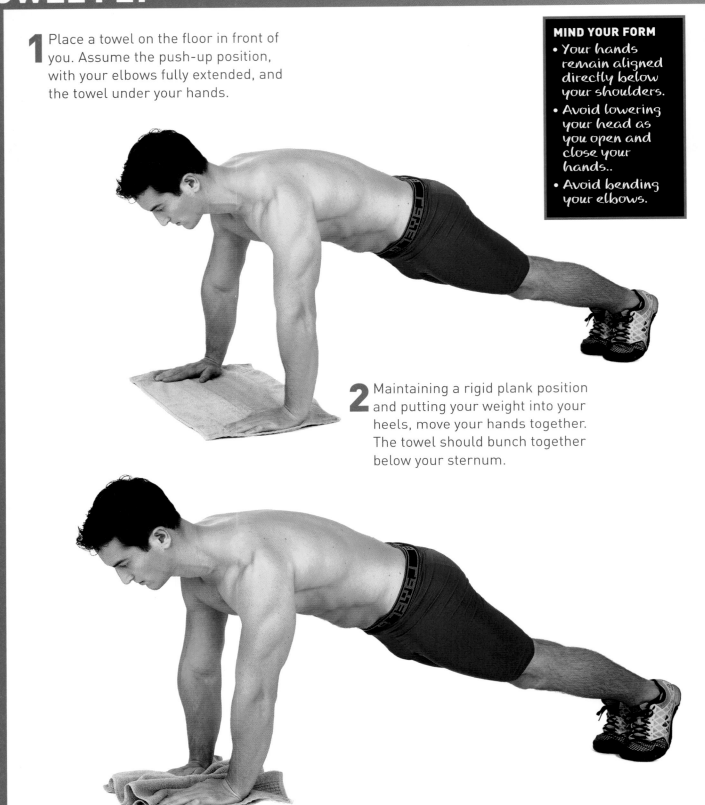

2 Maintaining a rigid plank position and putting your weight into your heels, move your hands together. The towel should bunch together below your sternum.

3 Straighten out the towel by pressing outward with your arms, returning to the starting position. Repeat 10 times.

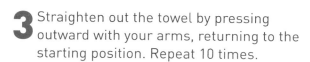

TYPE
• Strength

TARGET
• Chest
• Abdominals
• Shoulders
• Lower body
• Upper arms

EQUIPMENT
• Mat

MAJOR TARGETED MUSCLES

• deltoideus anterior
• deltoideus posterior
• pectoralis major
• pectoralis minor
• biceps brachii
• triceps brachii
• rectus femoris

ANNOTATION KEY

BOLD = MAJOR TARGETED MUSCLES
LIGHT = SECONDARY MUSCLES
* INDICATES DEEP MUSCLES

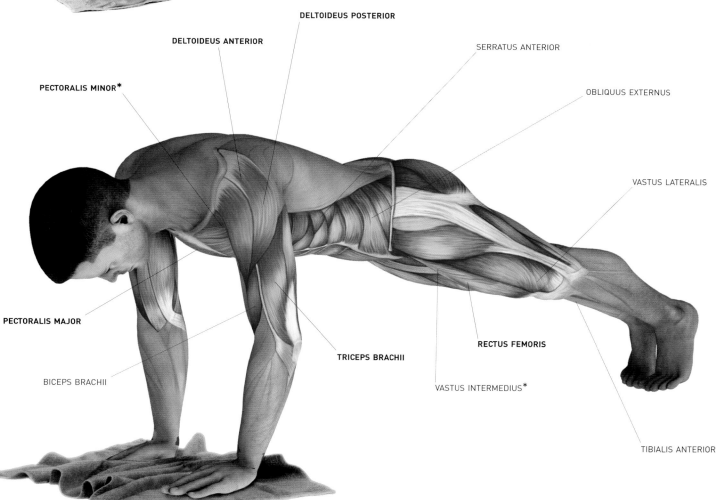

DELTOIDEUS POSTERIOR

DELTOIDEUS ANTERIOR

SERRATUS ANTERIOR

PECTORALIS MINOR*

OBLIQUUS EXTERNUS

VASTUS LATERALIS

PECTORALIS MAJOR

TRICEPS BRACHII

RECTUS FEMORIS

BICEPS BRACHII

VASTUS INTERMEDIUS*

TIBIALIS ANTERIOR

BURPEE

1 Stand with your feet hip-width apart and your arms above your head

2 Drop into a squat position, placing your hands on the floor.

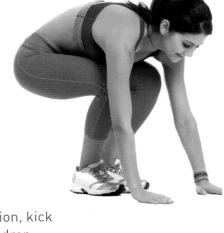

3 In one quick, explosive motion, kick your feet back to assume a drop position to perform a Push-Up .

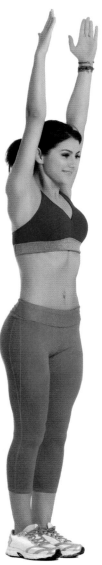

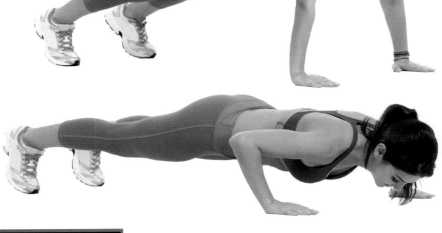

MIND YOUR FORM
- Make sure your chest touches the floor during step 3.
- Jump as high as you can as you rise from the squat.
- Avoid moving with floppy or jerky motions—your movement should be smooth and controlled.

4 In another quick motion, jump into the air, and return to the starting position.

5 Perform two sets, completing as many repetitions as possible in 60 seconds.

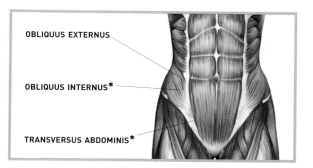

OBLIQUUS EXTERNUS
OBLIQUUS INTERNUS*
TRANSVERSUS ABDOMINIS*

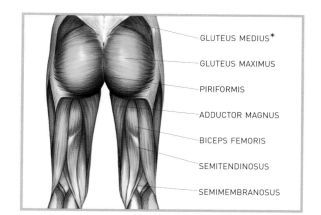

GLUTEUS MEDIUS*
GLUTEUS MAXIMUS
PIRIFORMIS
ADDUCTOR MAGNUS
BICEPS FEMORIS
SEMITENDINOSUS
SEMIMEMBRANOSUS

TYPE
• Cardio

TARGET
• Full body

EQUIPMENT
• None

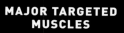

MAJOR TARGETED MUSCLES

• triceps brachii
• pectoralis major
• pectoralis minor
• coracobrachialis
• deltoideus anterior
• rectus abdominis
• transversus abdominis
• obliquus externus
• obliquus internus
• trapezius

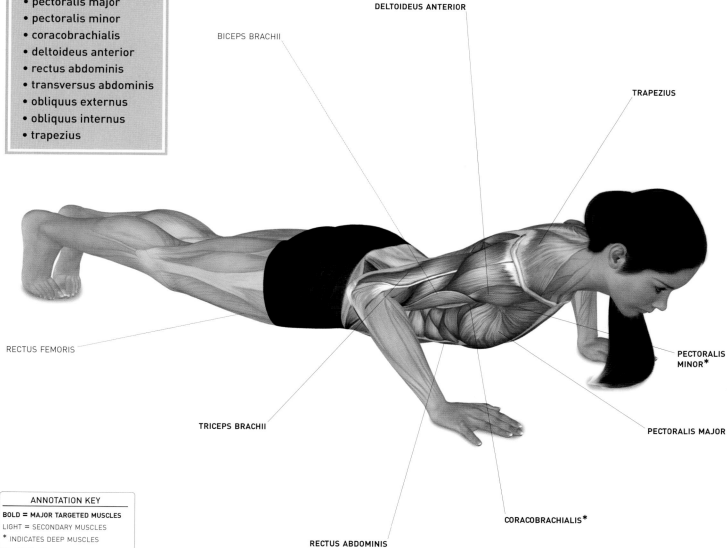

DELTOIDEUS ANTERIOR
BICEPS BRACHII
TRAPEZIUS
RECTUS FEMORIS
PECTORALIS MINOR*
TRICEPS BRACHII
PECTORALIS MAJOR
CORACOBRACHIALIS*
RECTUS ABDOMINIS

ANNOTATION KEY

BOLD = MAJOR TARGETED MUSCLES
LIGHT = SECONDARY MUSCLES
* INDICATES DEEP MUSCLES

MOUNTAIN CLIMBER

1 With your hands shoulder-width apart, place your palms on the floor, keeping your feet together and back straight. Push your body up until your arms are straight. Bring your right knee in toward your chest, and rest the ball of the foot on the floor for count 1.

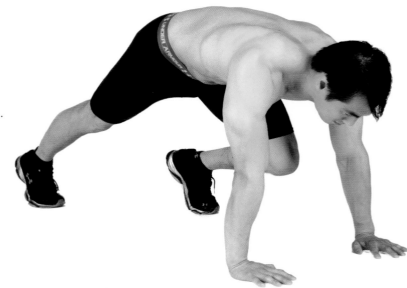

2 Jump, and bring your right knee to your chest for count 2.

MIND YOUR FORM
- Perform to a 4-count rhythm.
- Keep your back straight.
- Flare your hands out to ease shoulder stress.
- Avoid making small movements with your legs; Attempt to bring each knee to your chest for each count.
- Perform this exercise on a stable, nonslippery surface. Avoid exercise mats for his one—a surface like a hardwood floor will offer traction, but not shift under your feet or impede your movements.

3 Jump, and bring your left knee to your chest for count 3.

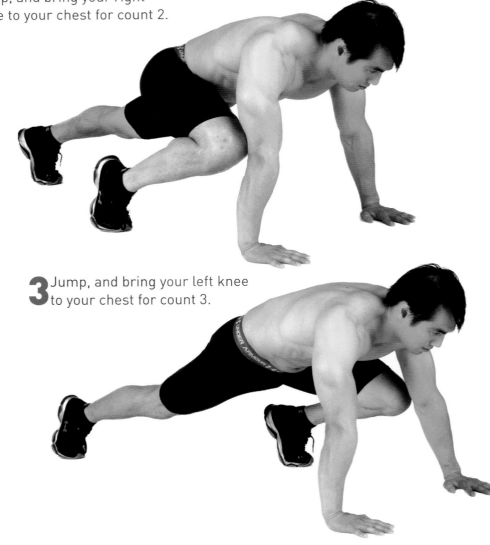

4 Jump, and bring your left knee to your chest for count 4. Continue alternating your feet as fast as you can safely go, keeping pace by counting 1-2-3-4. Each 1-to-4 count equals one repetition. Perform 10 reps.

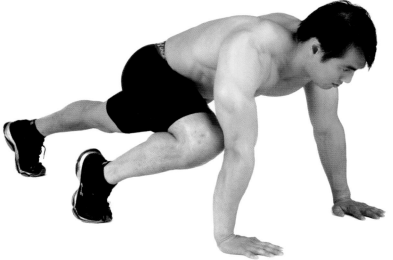

MAJOR TARGETED MUSCLES
• gluteus maximus
• vastus intermedius
• rectus femoris
• vastus lateralis
• gastrocnemius
• triceps brachii
• biceps brachii

TYPE
• Strength
• Cardio

TARGET
• Legs
• Arms

EQUIPMENT
• None

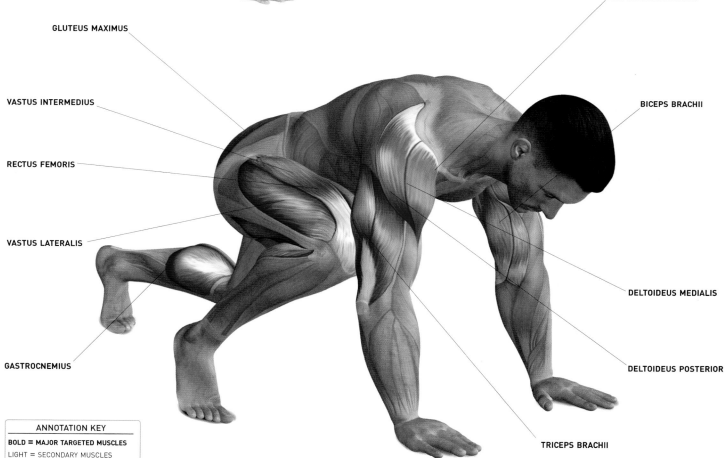

GLUTEUS MAXIMUS

VASTUS INTERMEDIUS

RECTUS FEMORIS

VASTUS LATERALIS

GASTROCNEMIUS

DELTOIDEUS ANTERIOR

BICEPS BRACHII

DELTOIDEUS MEDIALIS

DELTOIDEUS POSTERIOR

TRICEPS BRACHII

ANNOTATION KEY
BOLD = MAJOR TARGETED MUSCLES
LIGHT = SECONDARY MUSCLES
* INDICATES DEEP MUSCLES

REVERSE LUNGE

1 Stand with your hands on your hips and your feet shoulder-width apart.

2 Take a big step backward with your right foot, bending your knees as you do so and lowering your body, flexing your left knee and hip until your right leg is almost in contact with the floor.

3 When your front thigh is roughly parallel to the floor, push through your left heel, and bring your right foot forward to meet your left to the starting position.

4 Switch legs, and repeat on the other side, and then continue to alternate sides for a total of 10 repetitions on each leg. Perform two sets.

MIND YOUR FORM
- To fully engage your glutes, focus on pressing the heel of your front foot into the floor as you lift up.
- Keep your shoulders pressed downward.
- Keep your neck relaxed.
- Maintain upright form in your upper body as you lower and then raise your body.
- Keep your shoulders pressed downward.
- Avoid twisting either hip.
- Avoid hunching your shoulders.
- Avoid arching your back.

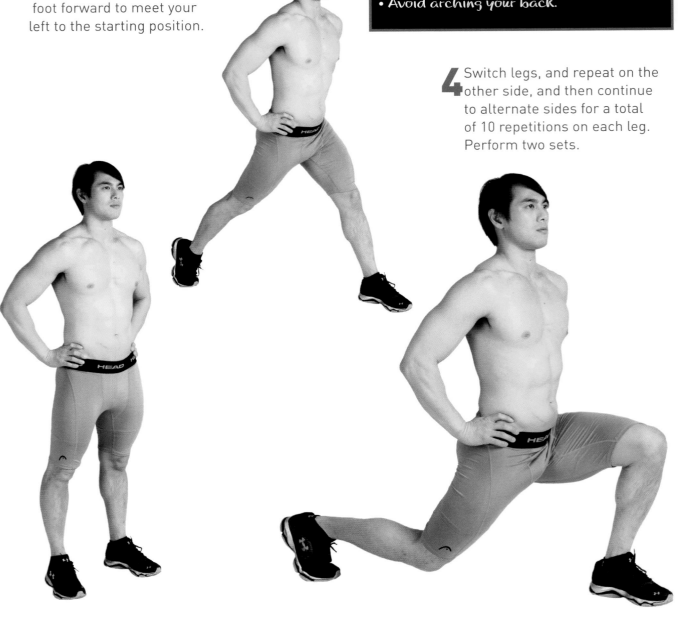

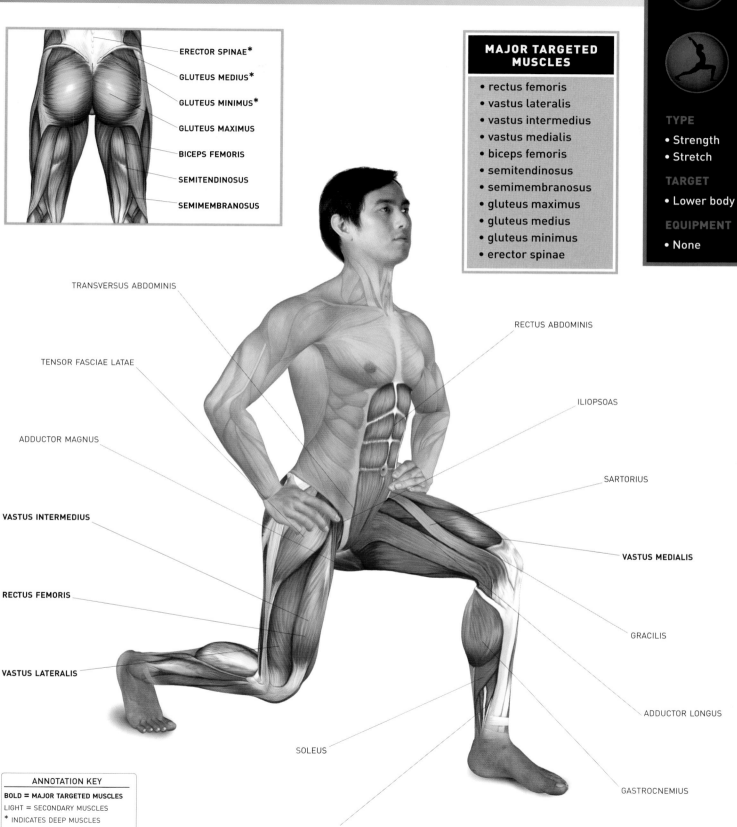

ERECTOR SPINAE*

GLUTEUS MEDIUS*

GLUTEUS MINIMUS*

GLUTEUS MAXIMUS

BICEPS FEMORIS

SEMITENDINOSUS

SEMIMEMBRANOSUS

MAJOR TARGETED MUSCLES

- rectus femoris
- vastus lateralis
- vastus intermedius
- vastus medialis
- biceps femoris
- semitendinosus
- semimembranosus
- gluteus maximus
- gluteus medius
- gluteus minimus
- erector spinae

TYPE
- Strength
- Stretch

TARGET
- Lower body

EQUIPMENT
- None

TRANSVERSUS ABDOMINIS

TENSOR FASCIAE LATAE

ADDUCTOR MAGNUS

VASTUS INTERMEDIUS

RECTUS FEMORIS

VASTUS LATERALIS

RECTUS ABDOMINIS

ILIOPSOAS

SARTORIUS

VASTUS MEDIALIS

GRACILIS

ADDUCTOR LONGUS

SOLEUS

GASTROCNEMIUS

ANNOTATION KEY

BOLD = MAJOR TARGETED MUSCLES

LIGHT = SECONDARY MUSCLES

* INDICATES DEEP MUSCLES

STEP-UP

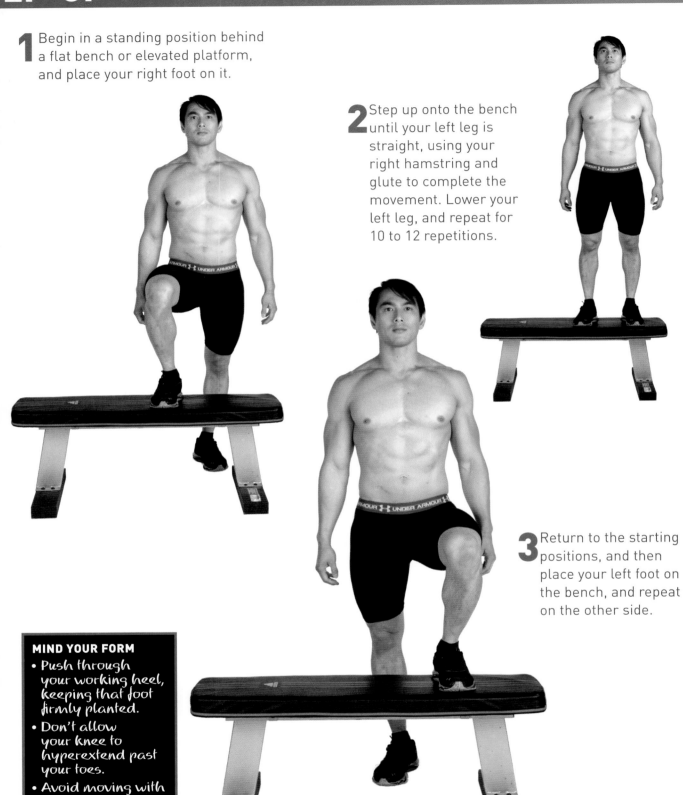

1 Begin in a standing position behind a flat bench or elevated platform, and place your right foot on it.

2 Step up onto the bench until your left leg is straight, using your right hamstring and glute to complete the movement. Lower your left leg, and repeat for 10 to 12 repetitions.

3 Return to the starting positions, and then place your left foot on the bench, and repeat on the other side.

MIND YOUR FORM
- Push through your working heel, keeping that foot firmly planted.
- Don't allow your knee to hyperextend past your toes.
- Avoid moving with excessive speed or momentum.

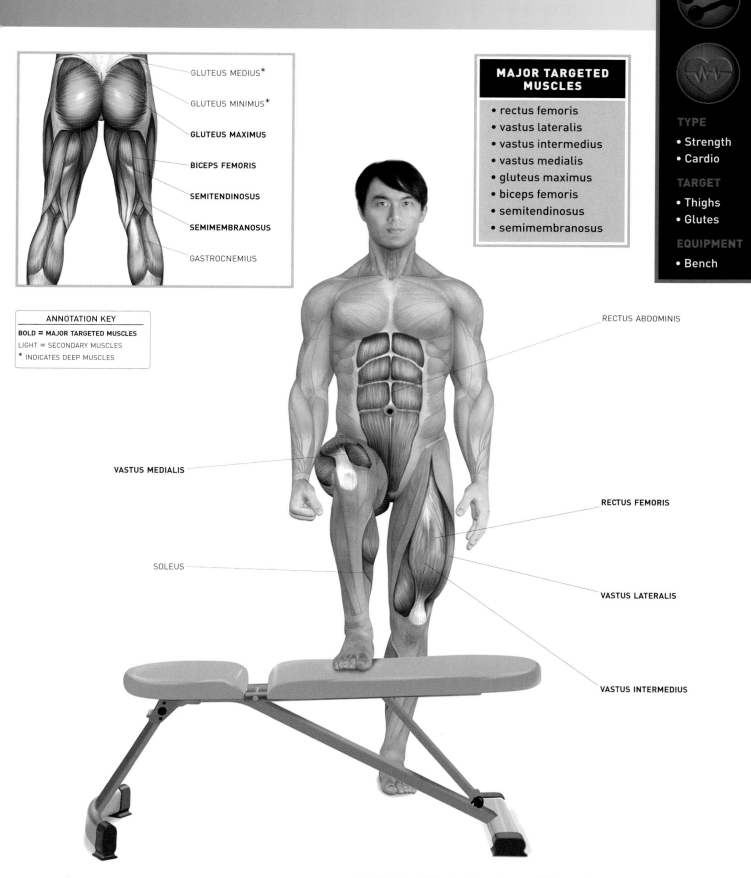

GLUTEUS MEDIUS*

GLUTEUS MINIMUS*

GLUTEUS MAXIMUS

BICEPS FEMORIS

SEMITENDINOSUS

SEMIMEMBRANOSUS

GASTROCNEMIUS

ANNOTATION KEY

BOLD = MAJOR TARGETED MUSCLES
LIGHT = SECONDARY MUSCLES
* INDICATES DEEP MUSCLES

MAJOR TARGETED MUSCLES

- rectus femoris
- vastus lateralis
- vastus intermedius
- vastus medialis
- gluteus maximus
- biceps femoris
- semitendinosus
- semimembranosus

TYPE
- Strength
- Cardio

TARGET
- Thighs
- Glutes

EQUIPMENT
- Bench

RECTUS ABDOMINIS

VASTUS MEDIALIS

RECTUS FEMORIS

SOLEUS

VASTUS LATERALIS

VASTUS INTERMEDIUS

INVERTED LEG EXTENSION

1 Begin in a standing position, feet shoulder-width apart, with your legs slightly bent and your arms above your head.

2 Bend forward at the waist while simultaneously spreading your arms out to your sides for balance and lifting your left leg behind you.

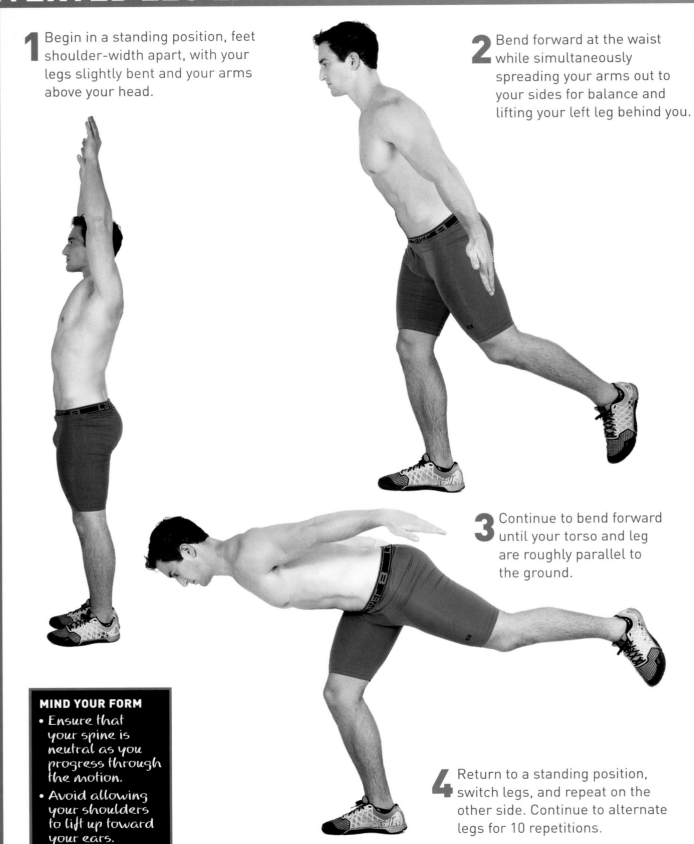

3 Continue to bend forward until your torso and leg are roughly parallel to the ground.

MIND YOUR FORM
- Ensure that your spine is neutral as you progress through the motion.
- Avoid allowing your shoulders to lift up toward your ears.

4 Return to a standing position, switch legs, and repeat on the other side. Continue to alternate legs for 10 repetitions.

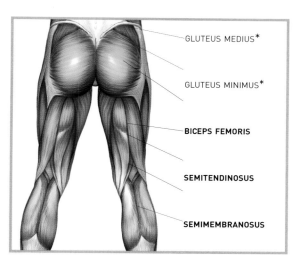

GLUTEUS MEDIUS*

GLUTEUS MINIMUS*

BICEPS FEMORIS

SEMITENDINOSUS

SEMIMEMBRANOSUS

MAJOR TARGETED MUSCLES

- triceps brachii
- rectus abdominis
- deltoideus posterior
- vastus medialis
- rectus femoris
- gastrocnemius
- biceps femoris
- semitendinosus
- semimembranosus
- gluteus maximus
- tractus iliotibialis

TYPE
- Strength

TARGET
- Full body

EQUIPMENT
- None

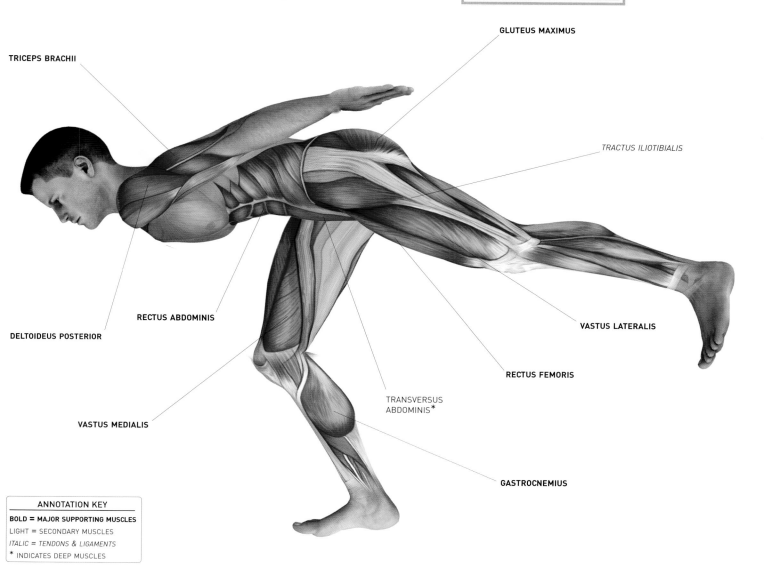

GLUTEUS MAXIMUS

TRICEPS BRACHII

TRACTUS ILIOTIBIALIS

RECTUS ABDOMINIS

DELTOIDEUS POSTERIOR

VASTUS LATERALIS

RECTUS FEMORIS

VASTUS MEDIALIS

TRANSVERSUS ABDOMINIS*

GASTROCNEMIUS

ANNOTATION KEY

BOLD = MAJOR SUPPORTING MUSCLES
LIGHT = SECONDARY MUSCLES
ITALIC = TENDONS & LIGAMENTS
* INDICATES DEEP MUSCLES

LATERAL STEP-OVER

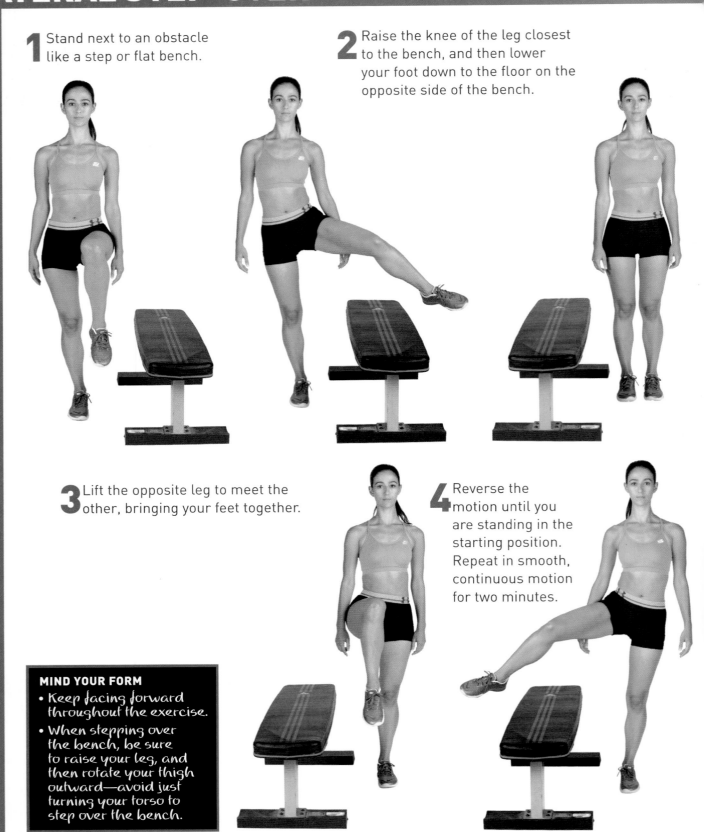

1 Stand next to an obstacle like a step or flat bench.

2 Raise the knee of the leg closest to the bench, and then lower your foot down to the floor on the opposite side of the bench.

3 Lift the opposite leg to meet the other, bringing your feet together.

4 Reverse the motion until you are standing in the starting position. Repeat in smooth, continuous motion for two minutes.

MIND YOUR FORM
- Keep facing forward throughout the exercise.
- When stepping over the bench, be sure to raise your leg, and then rotate your thigh outward—avoid just turning your torso to step over the bench.

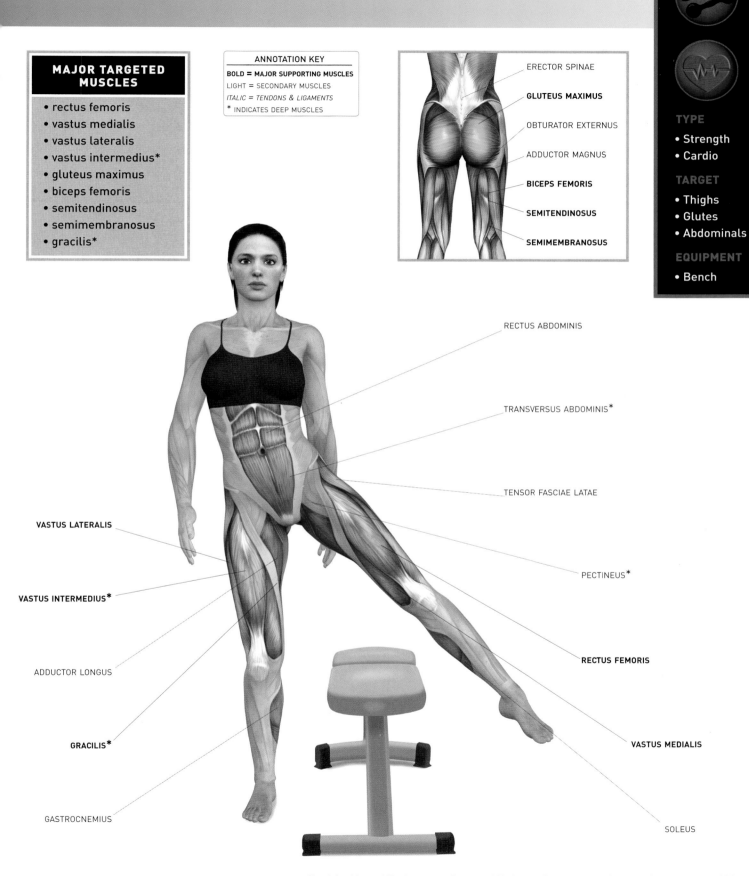

MAJOR TARGETED MUSCLES

- rectus femoris
- vastus medialis
- vastus lateralis
- vastus intermedius*
- gluteus maximus
- biceps femoris
- semitendinosus
- semimembranosus
- gracilis*

ANNOTATION KEY

BOLD = MAJOR SUPPORTING MUSCLES
LIGHT = SECONDARY MUSCLES
ITALIC = TENDONS & LIGAMENTS
* INDICATES DEEP MUSCLES

ERECTOR SPINAE

GLUTEUS MAXIMUS

OBTURATOR EXTERNUS

ADDUCTOR MAGNUS

BICEPS FEMORIS

SEMITENDINOSUS

SEMIMEMBRANOSUS

TYPE
- Strength
- Cardio

TARGET
- Thighs
- Glutes
- Abdominals

EQUIPMENT
- Bench

RECTUS ABDOMINIS

TRANSVERSUS ABDOMINIS*

TENSOR FASCIAE LATAE

VASTUS LATERALIS

VASTUS INTERMEDIUS*

ADDUCTOR LONGUS

PECTINEUS*

RECTUS FEMORIS

GRACILIS*

VASTUS MEDIALIS

GASTROCNEMIUS

SOLEUS

SIDE KICK

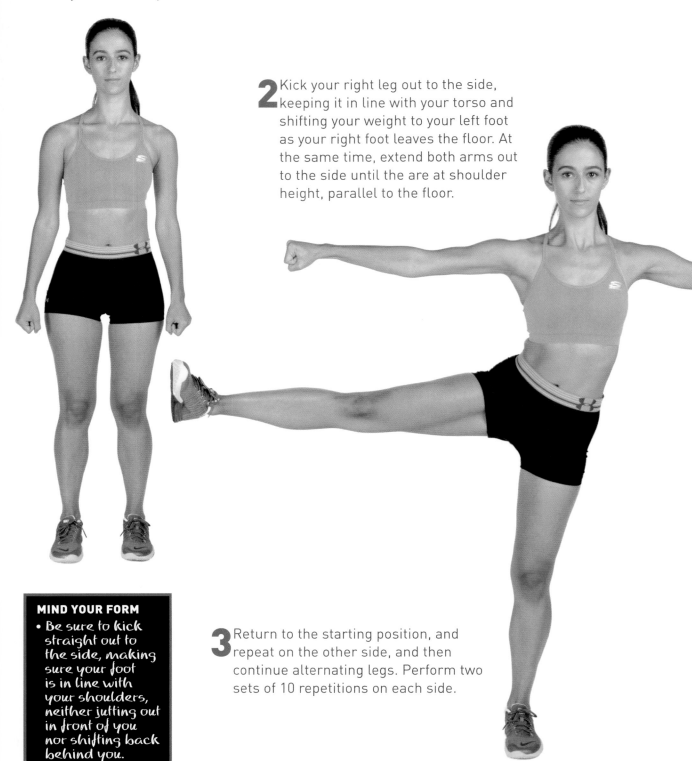

1 Stand with feet hip-width apart and your arms at your sides.

2 Kick your right leg out to the side, keeping it in line with your torso and shifting your weight to your left foot as your right foot leaves the floor. At the same time, extend both arms out to the side until the are at shoulder height, parallel to the floor.

MIND YOUR FORM
• Be sure to kick straight out to the side, making sure your foot is in line with your shoulders, neither jutting out in front of you nor shifting back behind you.

3 Return to the starting position, and repeat on the other side, and then continue alternating legs. Perform two sets of 10 repetitions on each side.

TYPE
- Cardio

TARGET
- Legs
- Upper back

EQUIPMENT
- None

MAJOR TARGETED MUSCLES

- supraspinatus
- teres minor
- rhomboideus
- gluteus medius
- gluteus maximus
- trapezius
- tensor fasciae latae
- sartorius
- rectus femoris
- vastus intermedius
- vastus lateralis
- iliopsoas

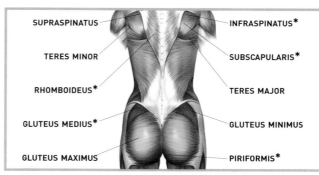

SUPRASPINATUS

TERES MINOR

RHOMBOIDEUS*

GLUTEUS MEDIUS*

GLUTEUS MAXIMUS

INFRASPINATUS*

SUBSCAPULARIS*

TERES MAJOR

GLUTEUS MINIMUS

PIRIFORMIS*

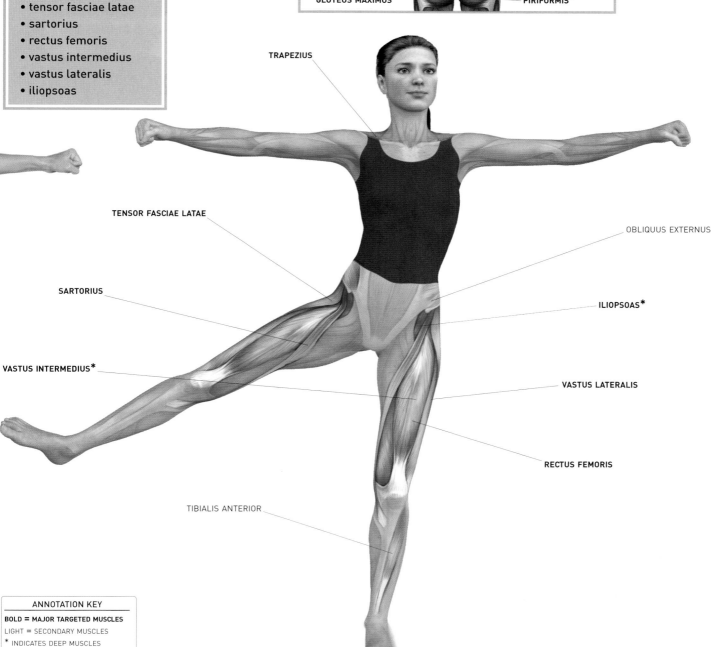

TRAPEZIUS

TENSOR FASCIAE LATAE

SARTORIUS

VASTUS INTERMEDIUS*

TIBIALIS ANTERIOR

OBLIQUUS EXTERNUS

ILIOPSOAS*

VASTUS LATERALIS

RECTUS FEMORIS

ANNOTATION KEY

BOLD = MAJOR TARGETED MUSCLES
LIGHT = SECONDARY MUSCLES
* INDICATES DEEP MUSCLES

SIDE-BEND PLANK

1 Lie on your right side with one arm supporting your torso, aligning the wrist under your shoulder. Place your left arm on top of your left leg. Your legs should be strongly squeezed together in adduction, with legs parallel and feet flexed. Draw your navel toward your spine.

MIND YOUR FORM
- Lift your hips high to take some weight off your upper body. Elongate your limbs as much as possible.
- Avoid allowing your shoulders to sink into their sockets or lift toward your ears

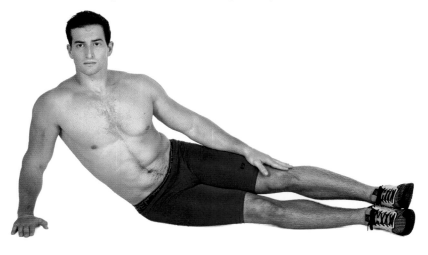

MAJOR TARGETED MUSCLES

- pectoralis major
- brachioradialis
- obliquus internus
- sartorius
- rectus femoris
- vastus medialis
- rectus abdominis
- transversus abdominis
- iliopsoas
- pectineus
- sartorius

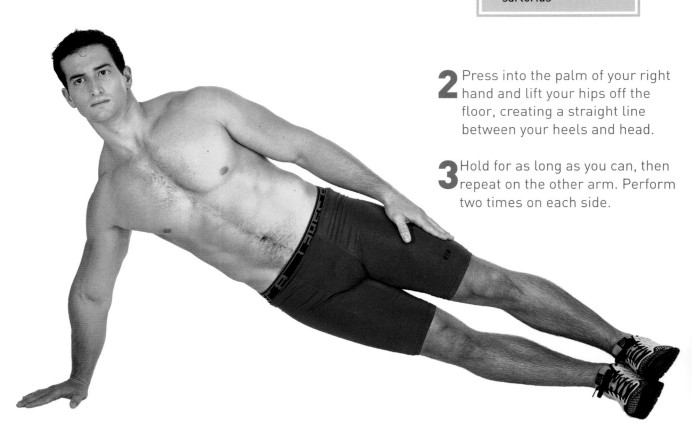

2 Press into the palm of your right hand and lift your hips off the floor, creating a straight line between your heels and head.

3 Hold for as long as you can, then repeat on the other arm. Perform two times on each side.

132

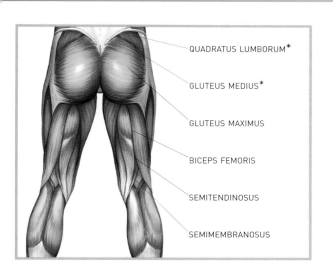

QUADRATUS LUMBORUM*

GLUTEUS MEDIUS*

GLUTEUS MAXIMUS

BICEPS FEMORIS

SEMITENDINOSUS

SEMIMEMBRANOSUS

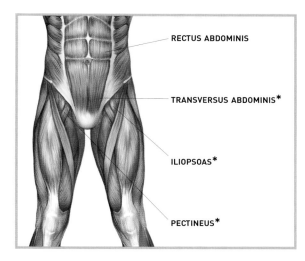

RECTUS ABDOMINIS

TRANSVERSUS ABDOMINIS*

ILIOPSOAS*

PECTINEUS*

TYPE
• Strength
TARGET
• Full body
EQUIPMENT
• None

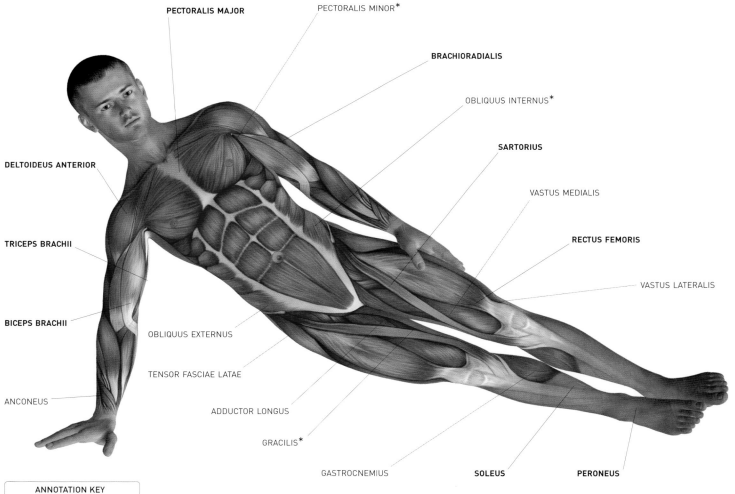

PECTORALIS MAJOR

PECTORALIS MINOR*

BRACHIORADIALIS

OBLIQUUS INTERNUS*

SARTORIUS

VASTUS MEDIALIS

DELTOIDEUS ANTERIOR

RECTUS FEMORIS

TRICEPS BRACHII

VASTUS LATERALIS

BICEPS BRACHII

OBLIQUUS EXTERNUS

TENSOR FASCIAE LATAE

ANCONEUS

ADDUCTOR LONGUS

GRACILIS*

GASTROCNEMIUS

SOLEUS

PERONEUS

ANNOTATION KEY

BOLD = MAJOR TARGETED MUSCLES

LIGHT = SECONDARY MUSCLES

* INDICATES DEEP MUSCLES

LEVEL THREE

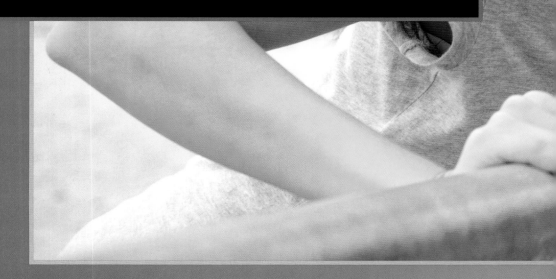

Congratulations on making it to Level Three. You are now ready to tackle the most advanced of the Healthy Heart workouts, building on the impressive achievements you've already accomplished.

Level Three workouts offer you a wide variety of demanding exercises, from fairly simple (but definately not easy) moves, like the Push-Up and Sit-Up, to multiphase ones, like Burpees (a favorite with grueling boot-camp style regimens). Also taken from boot camps are drills like the Four-Count Overhead, which you perform to a four-count, military beat. Just have fun and work hard—your heart will thank you

LEVEL THREE PROGRESS REPORT

WORKOUT	NAME	GOAL
A	Cardio-Strength Challenge	Improve full-body muscle strength and increase stamina and endurance
B	All-Around Challenge	Improve full-body muscle strength and increase stamina and endurance; increase flexibility and limberness. and develop better balance and coordination

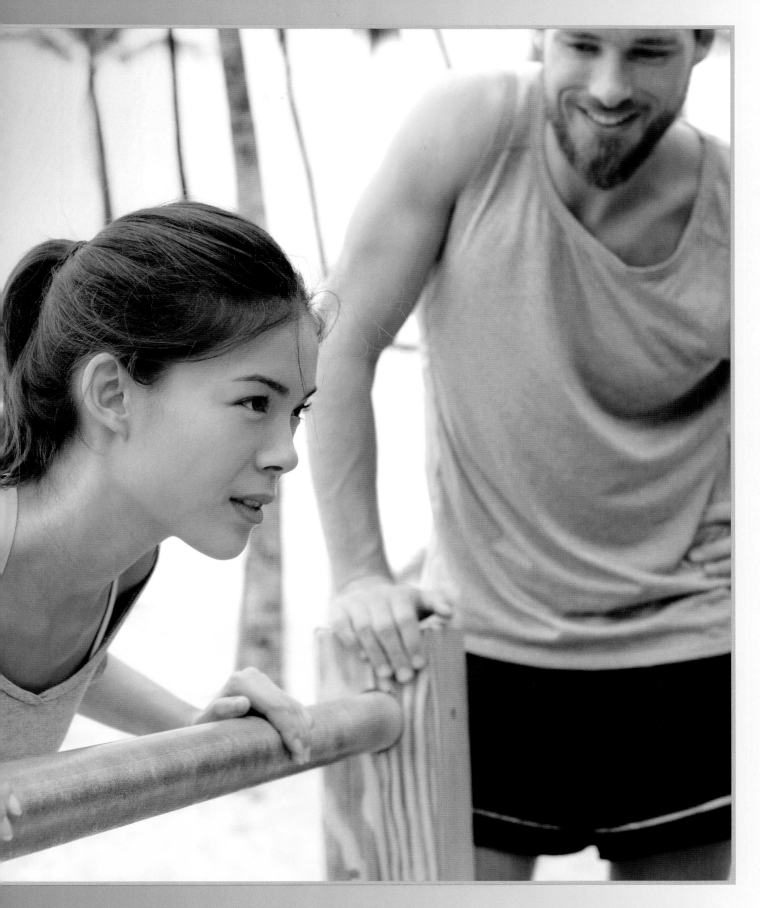

WORKOUT A

Cardio and Strength Challenge

Start your joint health regimen at the top, with a workout that targets your neck and shoulders. Whether you spend hours at your desk peering at a computer screen or toss heavy weights like a book-laden backpack across your shoulders every day, this area can too often hold a lot of tension. Try this beginner-level workout to help counteract that tightness and keep your shoulder and neck joints moving smoothly.

1. SPEED SKATER
(Pages 138–139)

Perform 10 repetitions.

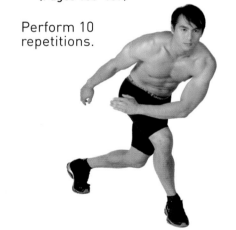

2. ROLL-UP
(Pages 140–141)

Perform two sets of five repetitions.

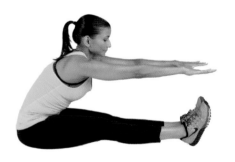

3. T-STABILIZATION
(Pages 142–143)

Perform 10 repetitions on each side.

4. SCISSORS
(Pages 144–145)

Perform 8 to 10 repetitions on each side.

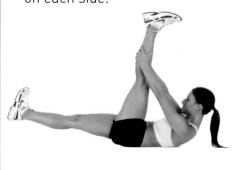

5. REACH-AND-TWIST WALKING LUNGE
(Pages 146–147)

Move forward for 15 steps.

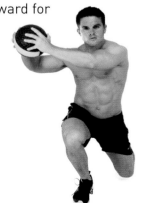

6. PUSH-UP
(Pages 148–149)

Perform two sets of 10 repetitions.

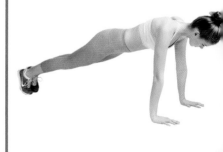

7. PLANK KNEE PULL-IN AND EXTEND
(Pages 150–151)

Perform 10 repetitions on each side.

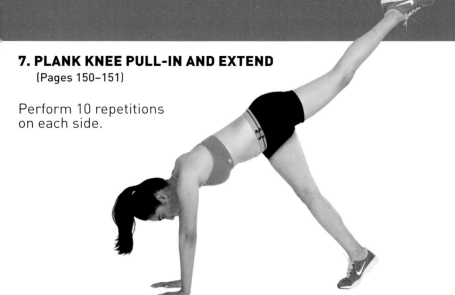

EQUIPMENT CHECKLIST
✗ Swiss ball
✔ medicine ball
✔ dumbbells
✗ barbell
✔ kettlebells
✔ mat
✗ chair
✗ bench
✗ aerobic step
✗ towel

8. SQUAT THRUST
(Pages 152–153)

Perform 15 repetitions.

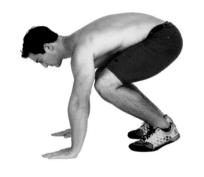

9. LUNGE WITH DUMBBELL UPRIGHT ROW
(Pages 154–155)

Perform 12 to 15 repetitions on each side.

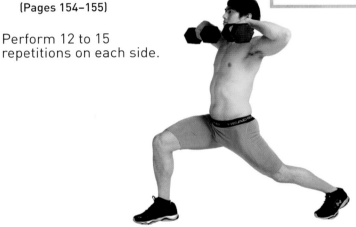

10. BOTTOMS-UP KETTLEBELL CLEAN
(Pages 156–157)

Perform 12 to 15 repetitions on each side.

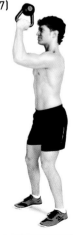

11. DOUBLE KETTLEBELL SNATCH
(Pages 158–159)

Perform 12 to 15 repetitions.

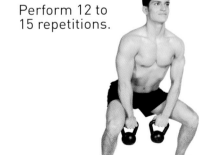

12. INCHWORM
(Pages 160–161)

Perform 5 to 10 repetitions.

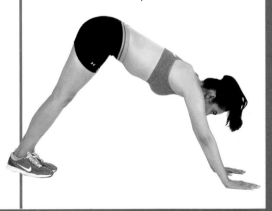

SPEED SKATER

1 Stand in a half-squat position, and place your left leg slightly behind your right.

2 Jump to your left as far as possible while swinging your arms toward the left. Land in a half-squat position with your right leg slightly behind your left.

MIND YOUR FORM
- Swing your arms together in the direction of the jump.
- Avoid moving your arms in any direction other than the direction of the jump.

3 Immediately jump back toward the right as far as possible, as if you were skating in long strides.

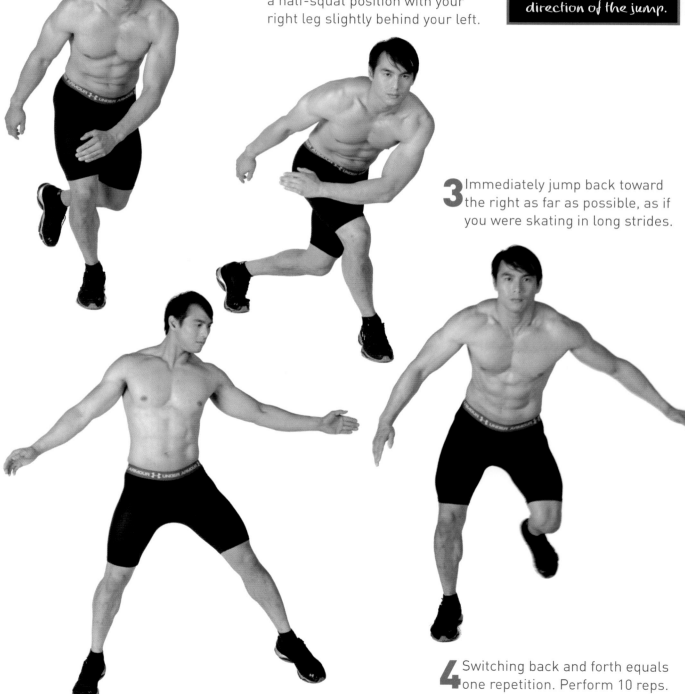

4 Switching back and forth equals one repetition. Perform 10 reps.

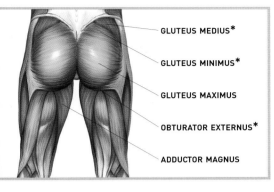

GLUTEUS MEDIUS*

GLUTEUS MINIMUS*

GLUTEUS MAXIMUS

OBTURATOR EXTERNUS*

ADDUCTOR MAGNUS

ANNOTATION KEY

BOLD = MAJOR SUPPORTING MUSCLES
LIGHT = SECONDARY MUSCLES
ITALIC = TENDONS & LIGAMENTS
* INDICATES DEEP MUSCLES

TYPE
• Cardio
TARGET
• Lower body
EQUIPMENT
• None

MAJOR TARGETED MUSCLES

- gluteus minimus
- gluteus maximus
- obturator externus
- adductor magnus
- gracilis
- tractus iliotibialis
- tensor fasciae latae
- pectineus
- adductor longus

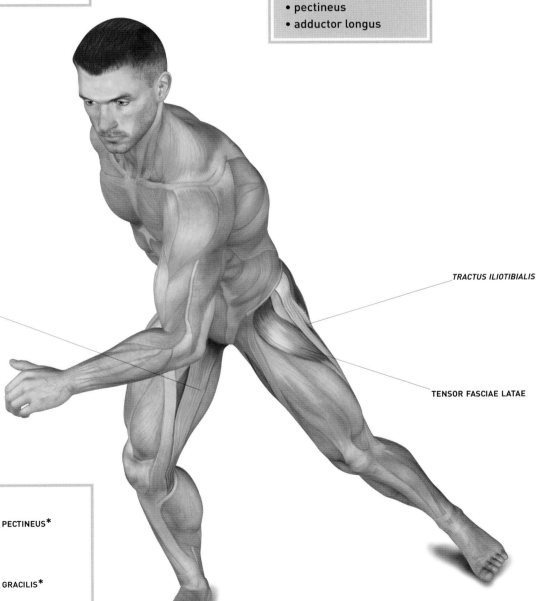

ADDUCTOR LONGUS

TRACTUS ILIOTIBIALIS

TENSOR FASCIAE LATAE

PECTINEUS*

GRACILIS*

ROLL-UP

1 Lie faceup on a mat, with your spine in neutral position and your ankles strongly flexed. Glide your shoulder blades down your back as you lift your arms overhead, extended slightly above the mat behind you. Press your shoulders and your rib cage downward.

MIND YOUR FORM
- Lead from your belly button.
- Avoid overusing your neck.
- Keep your abdominals fully engaged.
- Keep pressing your legs and heels into the floor for stabilization.
- Avoid momentum to roll up or down, bouncing, or otherwise compromising the fluid steadiness of the movements.

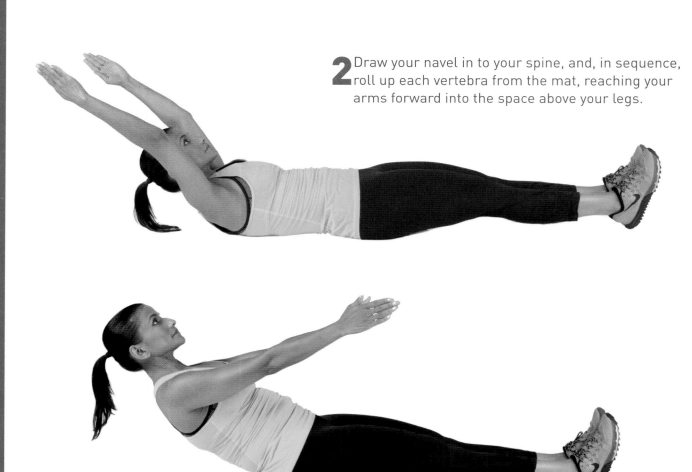

2 Draw your navel in to your spine, and, in sequence, roll up each vertebra from the mat, reaching your arms forward into the space above your legs.

3 Reverse the movement, rolling back down to the mat vertebra by vertebra, resisting the urge to lift your shoulders and collapse your chest. Perform two sets of five repetitions.

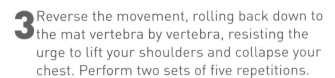

MAJOR TARGETED MUSCLES

- rectus abdominis
- erector spinae
- transversus abdominis
- iliopsoas
- serratus anterior
- obliquus externus
- obliquus internus
- erector spinae

TYPE
- Strength

TARGET
- Abdominals

EQUIPMENT
- Mat

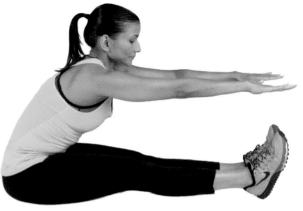

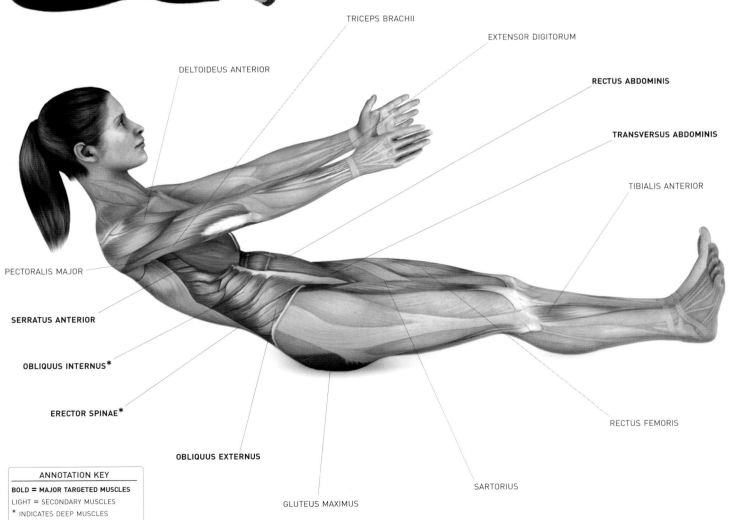

TRICEPS BRACHII

EXTENSOR DIGITORUM

DELTOIDEUS ANTERIOR

RECTUS ABDOMINIS

TRANSVERSUS ABDOMINIS

TIBIALIS ANTERIOR

PECTORALIS MAJOR

SERRATUS ANTERIOR

OBLIQUUS INTERNUS*

ERECTOR SPINAE*

RECTUS FEMORIS

OBLIQUUS EXTERNUS

SARTORIUS

GLUTEUS MAXIMUS

ANNOTATION KEY

BOLD = MAJOR TARGETED MUSCLES
LIGHT = SECONDARY MUSCLES
* INDICATES DEEP MUSCLES

T-STABILIZATION

1 Assume the drop position with your arms extended to full lockout, your fingers facing forward, your legs outstretched, and your body weight supported on your toes.

MIND YOUR FORM
- Engage your core, keeping your body in one straight line
- Avoid arching or bridging your lower back.

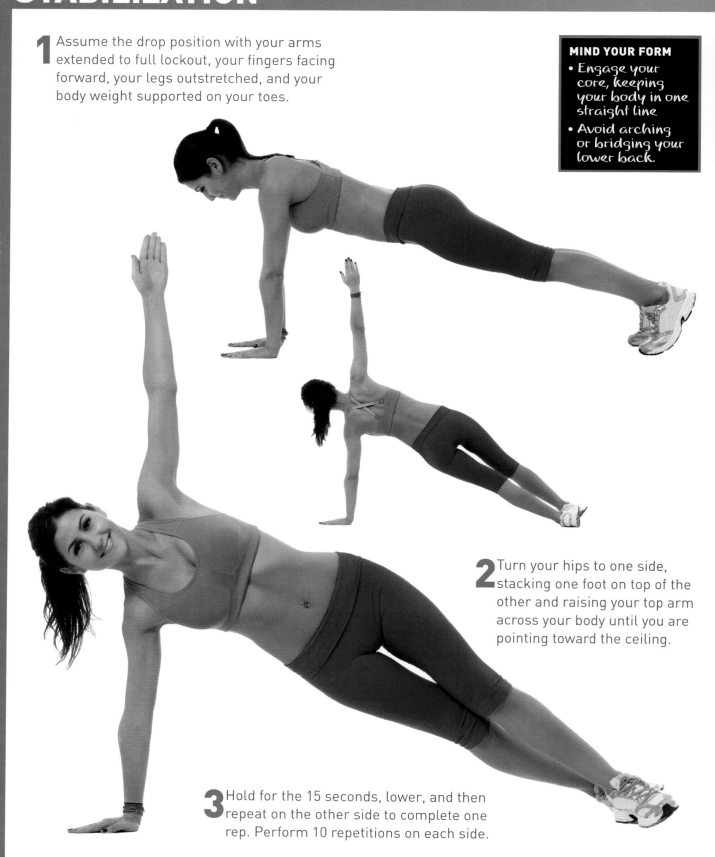

2 Turn your hips to one side, stacking one foot on top of the other and raising your top arm across your body until you are pointing toward the ceiling.

3 Hold for the 15 seconds, lower, and then repeat on the other side to complete one rep. Perform 10 repetitions on each side.

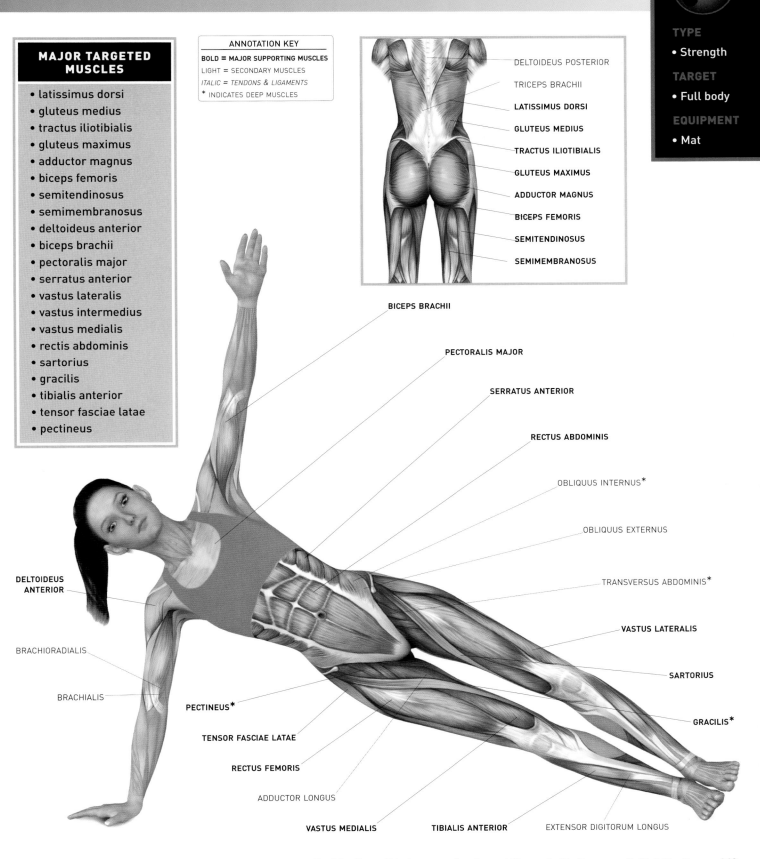

MAJOR TARGETED MUSCLES

- latissimus dorsi
- gluteus medius
- tractus iliotibialis
- gluteus maximus
- adductor magnus
- biceps femoris
- semitendinosus
- semimembranosus
- deltoideus anterior
- biceps brachii
- pectoralis major
- serratus anterior
- vastus lateralis
- vastus intermedius
- vastus medialis
- rectis abdominis
- sartorius
- gracilis
- tibialis anterior
- tensor fasciae latae
- pectineus

ANNOTATION KEY

BOLD = MAJOR SUPPORTING MUSCLES
LIGHT = SECONDARY MUSCLES
ITALIC = TENDONS & LIGAMENTS
* INDICATES DEEP MUSCLES

TYPE
- Strength

TARGET
- Full body

EQUIPMENT
- Mat

DELTOIDEUS POSTERIOR

TRICEPS BRACHII

LATISSIMUS DORSI

GLUTEUS MEDIUS

TRACTUS ILIOTIBIALIS

GLUTEUS MAXIMUS

ADDUCTOR MAGNUS

BICEPS FEMORIS

SEMITENDINOSUS

SEMIMEMBRANOSUS

BICEPS BRACHII

PECTORALIS MAJOR

SERRATUS ANTERIOR

RECTUS ABDOMINIS

OBLIQUUS INTERNUS*

OBLIQUUS EXTERNUS

TRANSVERSUS ABDOMINIS*

VASTUS LATERALIS

SARTORIUS

GRACILIS*

DELTOIDEUS ANTERIOR

BRACHIORADIALIS

BRACHIALIS

PECTINEUS*

TENSOR FASCIAE LATAE

RECTUS FEMORIS

ADDUCTOR LONGUS

VASTUS MEDIALIS

TIBIALIS ANTERIOR

EXTENSOR DIGITORUM LONGUS

SCISSORS

1 Lie on your back with your knees and feet lifted in tabletop position, your thighs making a 90-degree angle with your upper body, and your arms by your sides. Inhale, drawing in your abdominals.

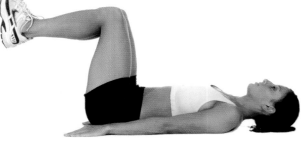

MIND YOUR FORM
- Keep your pelvis stabilized and your spine straight.
- Avoid overextending your raised leg

2 Stretching your right leg away from your body, raise your left leg towards your trunk. Hold your left calf with your hands, pulsing twice while keeping your shoulders down.

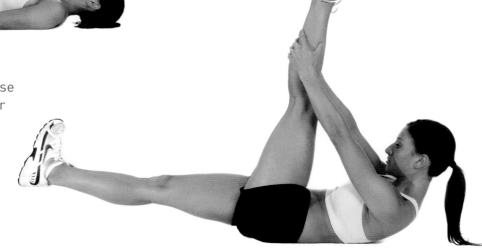

3 Switch your legs in the air, reaching for your right leg. Stabilize your pelvis and spine. Repeat sequence 8 to 10 times on each leg.

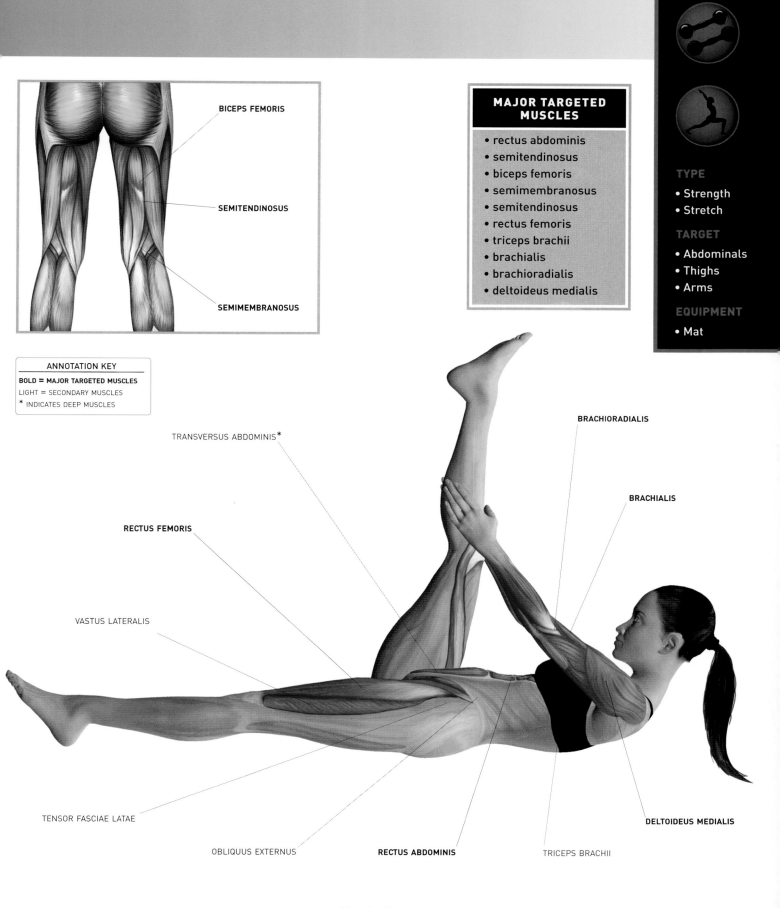

BICEPS FEMORIS

SEMITENDINOSUS

SEMIMEMBRANOSUS

MAJOR TARGETED MUSCLES

- rectus abdominis
- semitendinosus
- biceps femoris
- semimembranosus
- semitendinosus
- rectus femoris
- triceps brachii
- brachialis
- brachioradialis
- deltoideus medialis

TYPE
- Strength
- Stretch

TARGET
- Abdominals
- Thighs
- Arms

EQUIPMENT
- Mat

ANNOTATION KEY
BOLD = MAJOR TARGETED MUSCLES
LIGHT = SECONDARY MUSCLES
* INDICATES DEEP MUSCLES

TRANSVERSUS ABDOMINIS*

RECTUS FEMORIS

VASTUS LATERALIS

TENSOR FASCIAE LATAE

OBLIQUUS EXTERNUS

RECTUS ABDOMINIS

TRICEPS BRACHII

BRACHIORADIALIS

BRACHIALIS

DELTOIDEUS MEDIALIS

REACH-AND-TWIST WALKING LUNGE

1 Stand with feet roughly hip-width apart and your torso facing forward. Hold a weighted medicine ball in both hands.

2 Lunge your left foot forward. Begin to bend both knees, lowering your whole body into the lunge. At the same time, raise the medicine ball until it is over your left shoulder, held in both hands.

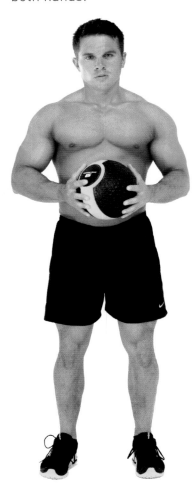

3 In a single motion, rise up to stand, bring the ball back to centre, and then perform the lunge and reach in the other direction.

4 Continue to lunge and move the ball from side to side as you walk forward. Continue for 15 steps.

MIND YOUR FORM
- Keep your torso facing forward.
- Keep your abdominal muscles engaged.
- Avoid hunching your shoulders or arching your back.

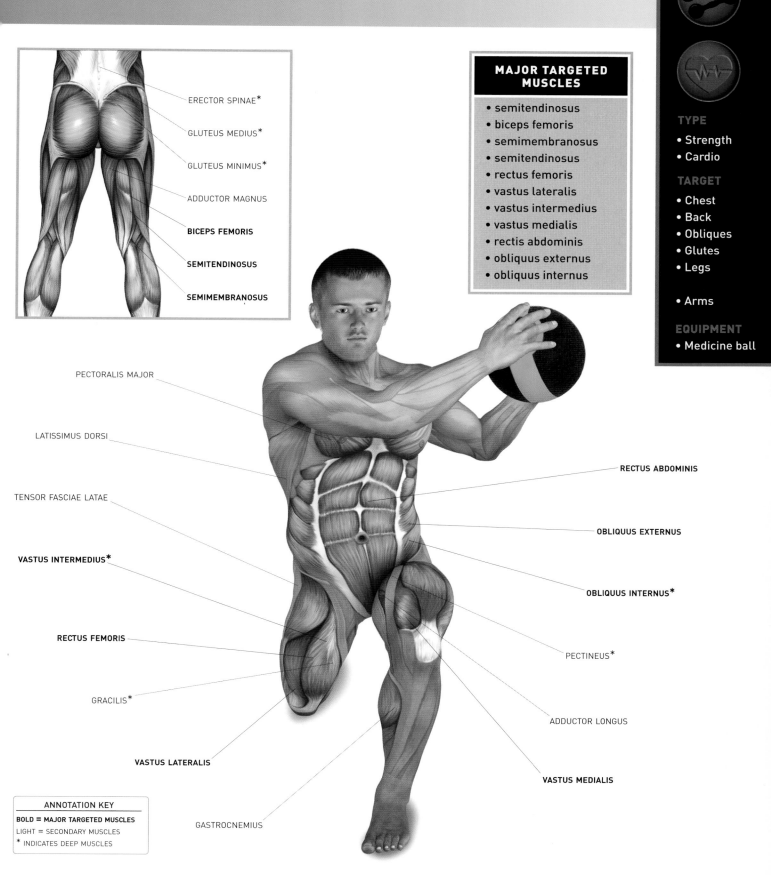

MAJOR TARGETED MUSCLES

- semitendinosus
- biceps femoris
- semimembranosus
- semitendinosus
- rectus femoris
- vastus lateralis
- vastus intermedius
- vastus medialis
- rectis abdominis
- obliquus externus
- obliquus internus

TYPE
- Strength
- Cardio

TARGET
- Chest
- Back
- Obliques
- Glutes
- Legs

- Arms

EQUIPMENT
- Medicine ball

ERECTOR SPINAE*

GLUTEUS MEDIUS*

GLUTEUS MINIMUS*

ADDUCTOR MAGNUS

BICEPS FEMORIS

SEMITENDINOSUS

SEMIMEMBRANOSUS

PECTORALIS MAJOR

LATISSIMUS DORSI

TENSOR FASCIAE LATAE

VASTUS INTERMEDIUS*

RECTUS FEMORIS

GRACILIS*

VASTUS LATERALIS

GASTROCNEMIUS

RECTUS ABDOMINIS

OBLIQUUS EXTERNUS

OBLIQUUS INTERNUS*

PECTINEUS*

ADDUCTOR LONGUS

VASTUS MEDIALIS

ANNOTATION KEY
BOLD = MAJOR TARGETED MUSCLES
LIGHT = SECONDARY MUSCLES
* INDICATES DEEP MUSCLES

PUSH-UP

1 From a kneeling position, place your hands firmly on the floor (or mat), directly under your shoulders or slightly wider than shoulder-width apart. Ground your toes into the floor to stabilize your lower half as you raise your body.

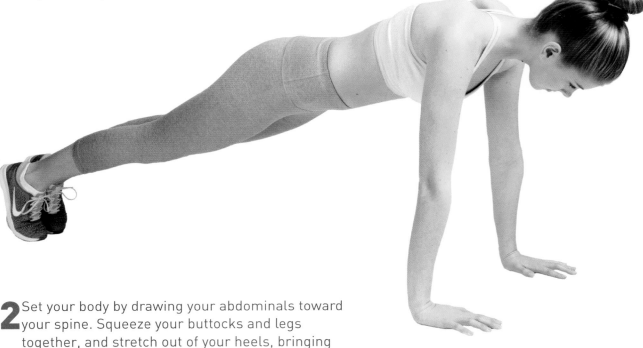

2 Set your body by drawing your abdominals toward your spine. Squeeze your buttocks and legs together, and stretch out of your heels, bringing your body into a straight line.

3 Bend your arms, and lower your torso until your chest touches the floor.

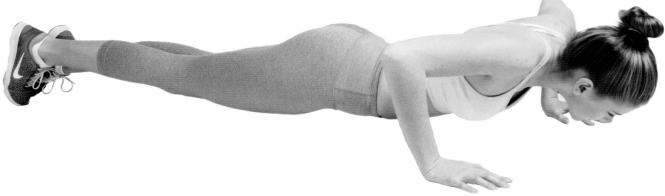

4 Straighten your arms to rise back to the starting position to complete the repetition. Perform two sets of 10 reps.

MIND YOUR FORM

- Slightly flare your hands outward to allow your elbows to go toward your hips as you lower yourself to the floor. This helps prevent shoulder tendonitis.
- If you cannot keep your back straight during the entire movement or you experience back pain, start this exercise on both knees and do a modified push-up.
- Don't point your elbows to the side during the down movement. This will place undue stress on your anterior deltoid muscles.
- Avoid pushing your hips into the air.

ANNOTATION KEY

BOLD = MAJOR TARGETED MUSCLES
LIGHT = SECONDARY MUSCLES
* INDICATES DEEP MUSCLES

MAJOR TARGETED MUSCLES

- triceps brachii
- pectoralis major
- pectoralis minor
- coracobrachialis
- deltoideus anterior
- rectus abdominis
- transversus abdominis
- obliquus externus
- obliquus internus
- trapezius

TYPE
- Strength

TARGET
- Shoulders
- Elbows
- Wrists

EQUIPMENT
- Mat

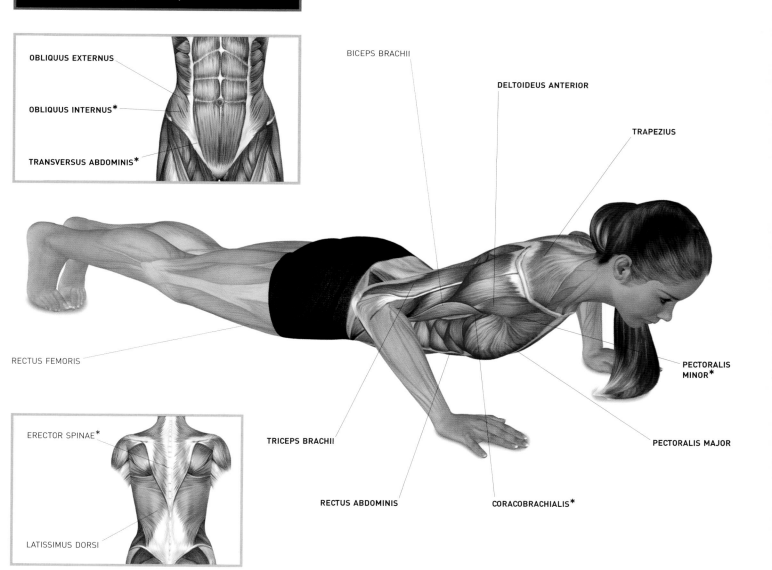

OBLIQUUS EXTERNUS

OBLIQUUS INTERNUS*

TRANSVERSUS ABDOMINIS*

BICEPS BRACHII

DELTOIDEUS ANTERIOR

TRAPEZIUS

RECTUS FEMORIS

PECTORALIS MINOR*

ERECTOR SPINAE*

TRICEPS BRACHII

PECTORALIS MAJOR

LATISSIMUS DORSI

RECTUS ABDOMINIS

CORACOBRACHIALIS*

PLANK KNEE PULL-IN AND EXTEND

1 Begin by assuming a plank position with your legs extended behind you and your hands positioned below your shoulders.

2 Draw your left knee into your chest while leaning forward and flexing your foot. Your right leg should be up on its toes.

MIND YOUR FORM
- Keep your body in a straight line throughout the exercise.
- Avoid bending the knee of the supporting leg.

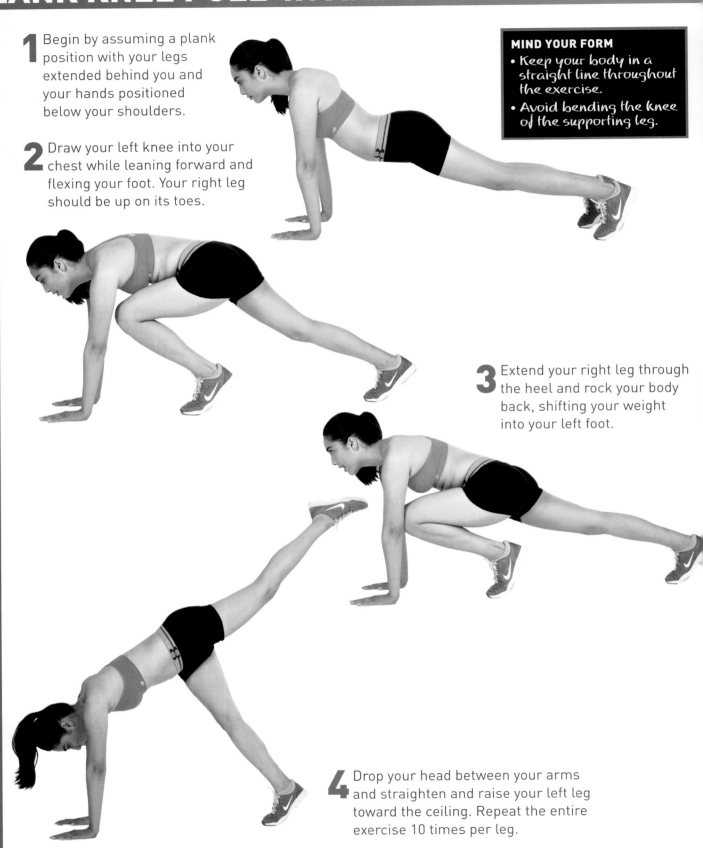

3 Extend your right leg through the heel and rock your body back, shifting your weight into your left foot.

4 Drop your head between your arms and straighten and raise your left leg toward the ceiling. Repeat the entire exercise 10 times per leg.

TYPE
• Strength

TARGET
• Full body

EQUIPMENT
• None

MAJOR TARGETED MUSCLES

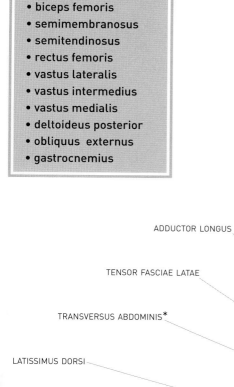

- quadratus lumborum
- gluteus medius
- gluteus minimus
- gluteus maximus
- semitendinosus
- biceps femoris
- semimembranosus
- semitendinosus
- rectus femoris
- vastus lateralis
- vastus intermedius
- vastus medialis
- deltoideus posterior
- obliquus externus
- gastrocnemius

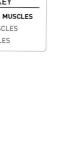

ANNOTATION KEY

BOLD = MAJOR TARGETED MUSCLES
LIGHT = SECONDARY MUSCLES
* INDICATES DEEP MUSCLES

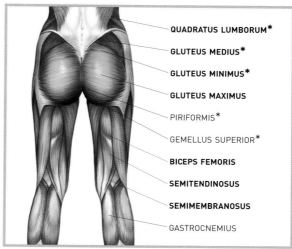

- **QUADRATUS LUMBORUM***
- **GLUTEUS MEDIUS***
- **GLUTEUS MINIMUS***
- **GLUTEUS MAXIMUS**
- PIRIFORMIS*
- GEMELLUS SUPERIOR*
- **BICEPS FEMORIS**
- **SEMITENDINOSUS**
- **SEMIMEMBRANOSUS**
- GASTROCNEMIUS

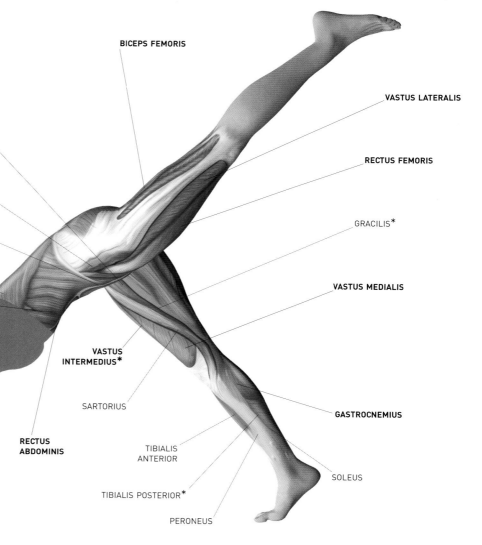

- **BICEPS FEMORIS**
- ADDUCTOR LONGUS
- TENSOR FASCIAE LATAE
- TRANSVERSUS ABDOMINIS*
- LATISSIMUS DORSI
- **OBLIQUUS EXTERNUS**
- TERES MAJOR
- **DELTOIDEUS POSTERIOR**
- **VASTUS LATERALIS**
- **RECTUS FEMORIS**
- GRACILIS*
- **VASTUS MEDIALIS**
- **VASTUS INTERMEDIUS***
- SARTORIUS
- RECTUS ABDOMINIS
- TIBIALIS ANTERIOR
- TIBIALIS POSTERIOR*
- PERONEUS
- **GASTROCNEMIUS**
- SOLEUS

SQUAT THRUST

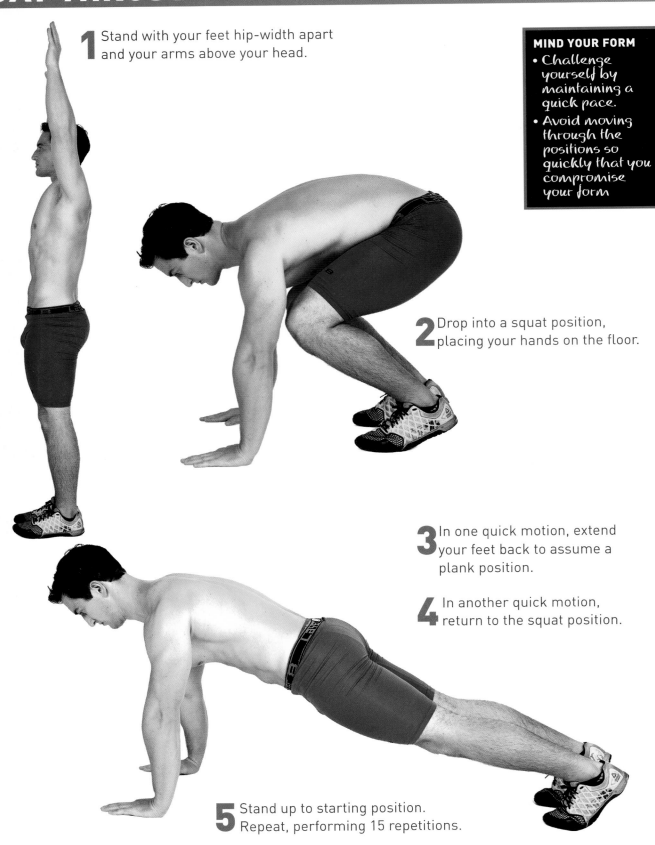

1 Stand with your feet hip-width apart and your arms above your head.

MIND YOUR FORM
- Challenge yourself by maintaining a quick pace.
- Avoid moving through the positions so quickly that you compromise your form

2 Drop into a squat position, placing your hands on the floor.

3 In one quick motion, extend your feet back to assume a plank position.

4 In another quick motion, return to the squat position.

5 Stand up to starting position. Repeat, performing 15 repetitions.

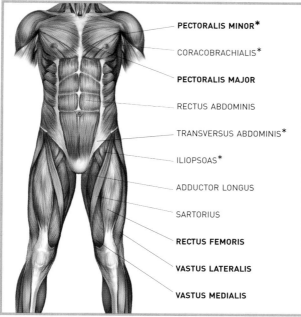

PECTORALIS MINOR*

CORACOBRACHIALIS*

PECTORALIS MAJOR

RECTUS ABDOMINIS

TRANSVERSUS ABDOMINIS*

ILIOPSOAS*

ADDUCTOR LONGUS

SARTORIUS

RECTUS FEMORIS

VASTUS LATERALIS

VASTUS MEDIALIS

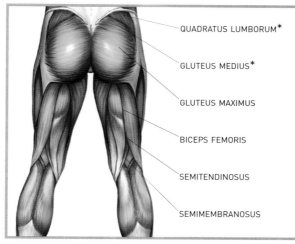

QUADRATUS LUMBORUM*

GLUTEUS MEDIUS*

GLUTEUS MAXIMUS

BICEPS FEMORIS

SEMITENDINOSUS

SEMIMEMBRANOSUS

ANNOTATION KEY

BOLD = MAJOR TARGETED MUSCLES
LIGHT = SECONDARY MUSCLES
* INDICATES DEEP MUSCLES

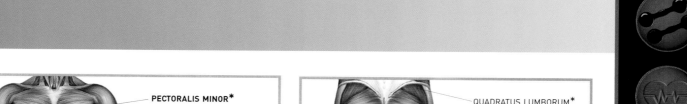

TYPE
- Strength
- Cardio

TARGET
- Chest
- Shoulders
- Glutes
- Legs

EQUIPMENT
- None

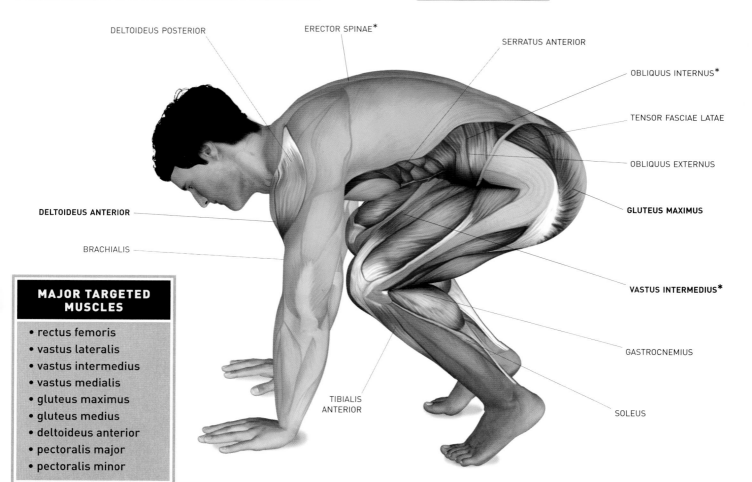

DELTOIDEUS POSTERIOR

ERECTOR SPINAE*

SERRATUS ANTERIOR

OBLIQUUS INTERNUS*

TENSOR FASCIAE LATAE

OBLIQUUS EXTERNUS

GLUTEUS MAXIMUS

DELTOIDEUS ANTERIOR

BRACHIALIS

VASTUS INTERMEDIUS*

GASTROCNEMIUS

TIBIALIS ANTERIOR

SOLEUS

MAJOR TARGETED MUSCLES

- rectus femoris
- vastus lateralis
- vastus intermedius
- vastus medialis
- gluteus maximus
- gluteus medius
- deltoideus anterior
- pectoralis major
- pectoralis minor

LUNGE WITH DUMBBELL UPRIGHT ROW

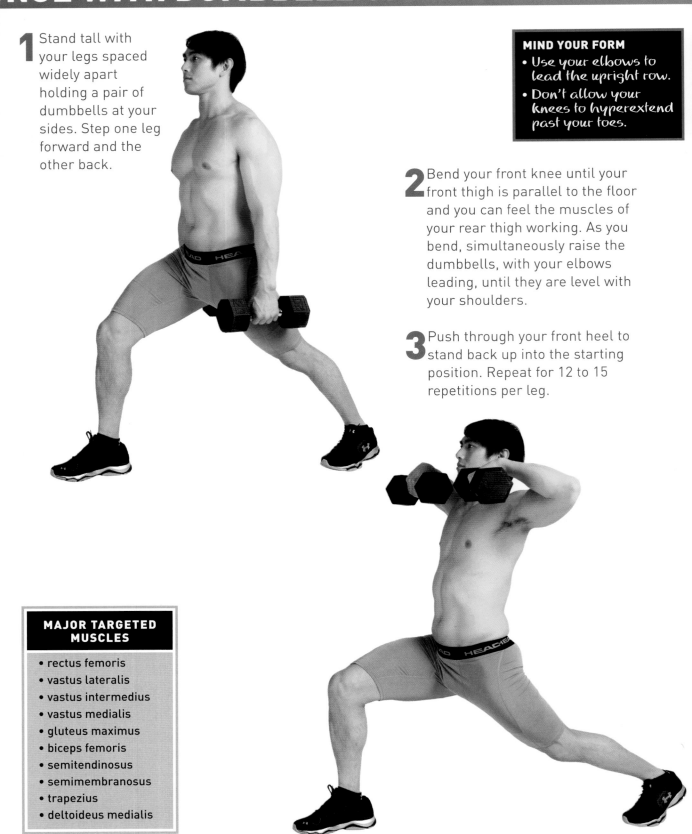

1 Stand tall with your legs spaced widely apart holding a pair of dumbbells at your sides. Step one leg forward and the other back.

MIND YOUR FORM
- Use your elbows to lead the upright row.
- Don't allow your knees to hyperextend past your toes.

2 Bend your front knee until your front thigh is parallel to the floor and you can feel the muscles of your rear thigh working. As you bend, simultaneously raise the dumbbells, with your elbows leading, until they are level with your shoulders.

3 Push through your front heel to stand back up into the starting position. Repeat for 12 to 15 repetitions per leg.

MAJOR TARGETED MUSCLES

- rectus femoris
- vastus lateralis
- vastus intermedius
- vastus medialis
- gluteus maximus
- biceps femoris
- semitendinosus
- semimembranosus
- trapezius
- deltoideus medialis

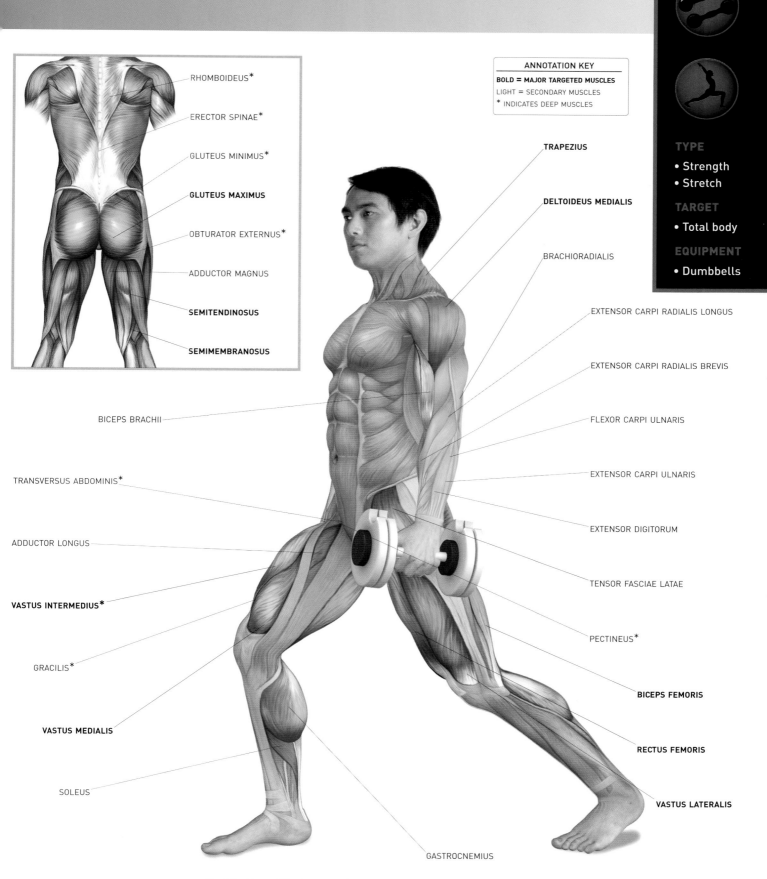

ANNOTATION KEY

BOLD = MAJOR TARGETED MUSCLES
LIGHT = SECONDARY MUSCLES
* INDICATES DEEP MUSCLES

RHOMBOIDEUS*

ERECTOR SPINAE*

GLUTEUS MINIMUS*

GLUTEUS MAXIMUS

OBTURATOR EXTERNUS*

ADDUCTOR MAGNUS

SEMITENDINOSUS

SEMIMEMBRANOSUS

TRAPEZIUS

DELTOIDEUS MEDIALIS

BRACHIORADIALIS

EXTENSOR CARPI RADIALIS LONGUS

EXTENSOR CARPI RADIALIS BREVIS

FLEXOR CARPI ULNARIS

EXTENSOR CARPI ULNARIS

EXTENSOR DIGITORUM

TENSOR FASCIAE LATAE

PECTINEUS*

BICEPS FEMORIS

RECTUS FEMORIS

VASTUS LATERALIS

BICEPS BRACHII

TRANSVERSUS ABDOMINIS*

ADDUCTOR LONGUS

VASTUS INTERMEDIUS*

GRACILIS*

VASTUS MEDIALIS

SOLEUS

GASTROCNEMIUS

TYPE
• Strength
• Stretch
TARGET
• Total body
EQUIPMENT
• Dumbbells

Healthy Heart Workouts • Cardio and Strength Challenge • Lunge with Dumbbell Upright Row • 155

BOTTOMS-UP KETTLEBELL CLEAN

1 Stand upright, with your feet shoulder-width apart, holding a kettlebell in your left hand.

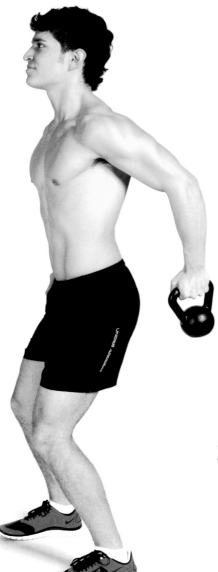

2 Swing the kettlebell backward, then bring it forward and above your head forcefully, squeezing the handle as you do so.

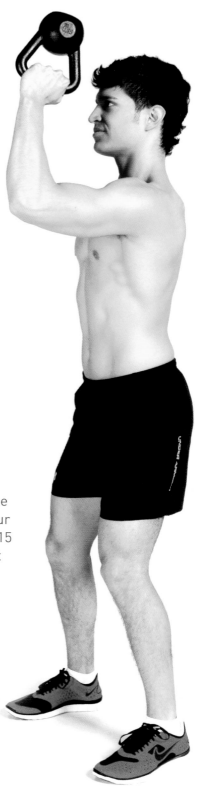

3 Once your upper arm is parallel to the floor, hold the position, and then lower your arm again. Complete 12 to 15 repetitions, and then repeat with the other arm.

MIND YOUR FORM
• Keep your upper arm close to your body as if you were tucking a purse or newspaper under your arm.

MAJOR TARGETED MUSCLES

• extensor digitorum
• anconeus
• flexor digitorum
• flexor carpi radialis
• deltoideus anterior
• deltoideus medialis
• deltoideus posterior
• triceps brachii
• biceps brachii
• pectoralis major
• pectoralis minor
• palmaris longus
• pronator teres

EXTENSOR DIGITORUM

ANCONEUS

TRICEPS BRACHII

DELTOIDEUS ANTERIOR

DELTOIDEUS MEDIALIS

BICEPS BRACHII

PECTORALIS MINOR*

PECTORALIS MAJOR

PALMARIS LONGUS

PRONATOR TERES

FLEXOR DIGITORUM*

FLEXOR CARPI ULNARIS

TYPE
• Strength
• Cardio

TARGET
• Chest
• Shoulders
• Arms

EQUIPMENT
• Kettlebells

ANNOTATION KEY

BOLD = MAJOR TARGETED MUSCLES
LIGHT = SECONDARY MUSCLES
* INDICATES DEEP MUSCLES

DOUBLE KETTLEBELL SNATCH

1 Stand with your feet a little more than shoulder-width apart, holding a pair of kettlebells at your sides.

2 Squat down, leaning forward slightly and sticking out your buttocks. Bring your arms between your legs, so that the kettlebells are next to your inner thighs.

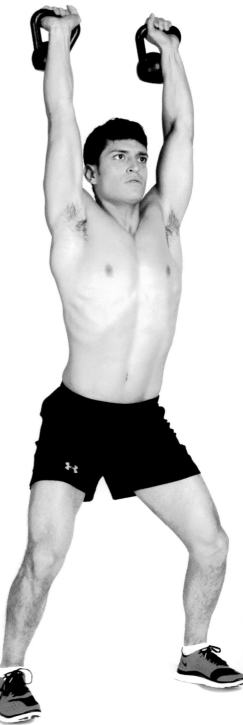
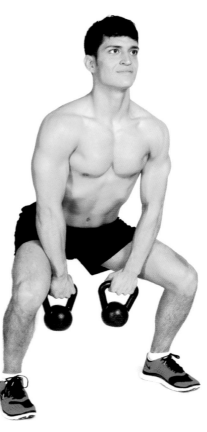
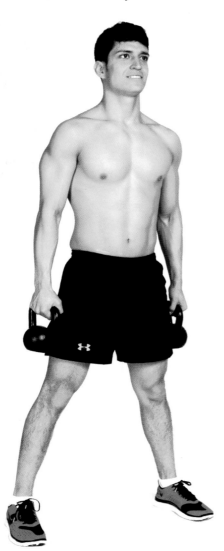

MIND YOUR FORM

• As you swing the bell upward, shrug your shoulders backward, which will pull the weights closer to your body, making then feel lighter when they reach the apex.

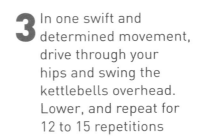

3 In one swift and determined movement, drive through your hips and swing the kettlebells overhead. Lower, and repeat for 12 to 15 repetitions

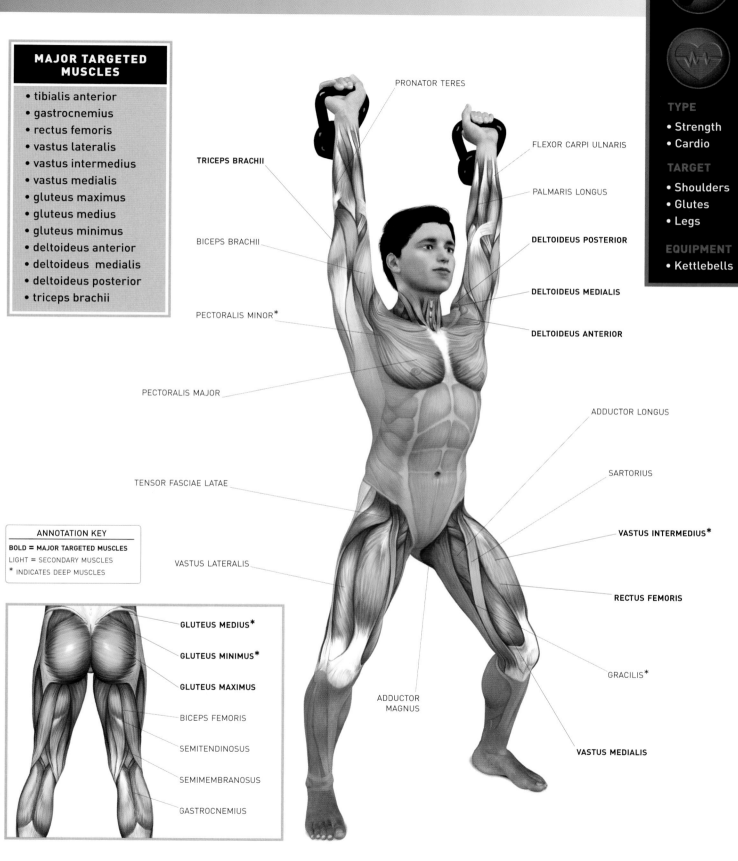

MAJOR TARGETED MUSCLES

- tibialis anterior
- gastrocnemius
- rectus femoris
- vastus lateralis
- vastus intermedius
- vastus medialis
- gluteus maximus
- gluteus medius
- gluteus minimus
- deltoideus anterior
- deltoideus medialis
- deltoideus posterior
- triceps brachii

TYPE
- Strength
- Cardio

TARGET
- Shoulders
- Glutes
- Legs

EQUIPMENT
- Kettlebells

PRONATOR TERES

FLEXOR CARPI ULNARIS

PALMARIS LONGUS

TRICEPS BRACHII

BICEPS BRACHII

DELTOIDEUS POSTERIOR

DELTOIDEUS MEDIALIS

PECTORALIS MINOR*

DELTOIDEUS ANTERIOR

PECTORALIS MAJOR

ADDUCTOR LONGUS

SARTORIUS

TENSOR FASCIAE LATAE

VASTUS INTERMEDIUS*

RECTUS FEMORIS

ANNOTATION KEY
BOLD = MAJOR TARGETED MUSCLES
LIGHT = SECONDARY MUSCLES
* INDICATES DEEP MUSCLES

VASTUS LATERALIS

GRACILIS*

ADDUCTOR MAGNUS

VASTUS MEDIALIS

GLUTEUS MEDIUS*

GLUTEUS MINIMUS*

GLUTEUS MAXIMUS

BICEPS FEMORIS

SEMITENDINOSUS

SEMIMEMBRANOSUS

GASTROCNEMIUS

INCHWORM

1 Begin in a standing position.

2 Bend forward, touching your fingertips to the floor.

3 Start walking your hands forward.

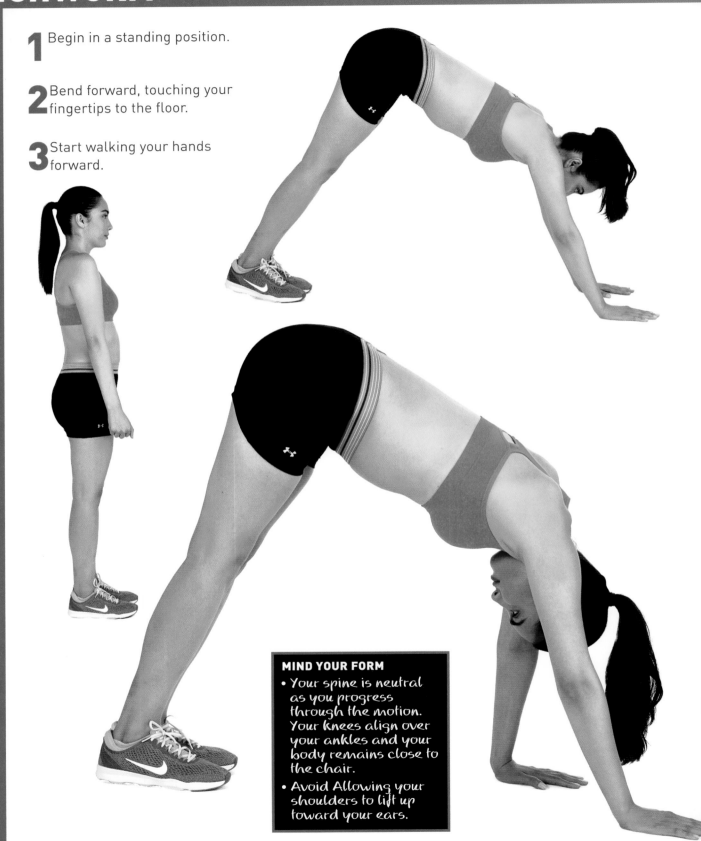

MIND YOUR FORM

- Your spine is neutral as you progress through the motion. Your knees align over your ankles and your body remains close to the chair.
- Avoid Allowing your shoulders to lift up toward your ears.

160

4 Continue walking your hands forward until you are in a push-up position, while keeping your legs straight.

5 Slowly walk your feet back to your hands, returning to the starting position. Repeat for 5 to 10 repetitions.

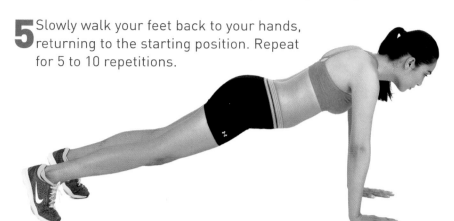

MAJOR TARGETED MUSCLES

- tibialis anterior
- deltoideus posterior
- deltoideus medialis
- deltoideus anterior
- latissimus dorsi
- serratus anterior
- transversus abdominis
- biceps femoris
- semitendinosus
- semimembranosus
- gluteus maximus
- erector spinae
- rectus abdominis
- pectoralis major
- pectoralis minor

TYPE
- Strength

TARGET
- Full body

EQUIPMENT
- None

ANNOTATION KEY
BOLD = MAJOR TARGETED MUSCLES
LIGHT = SECONDARY MUSCLES
* INDICATES DEEP MUSCLES

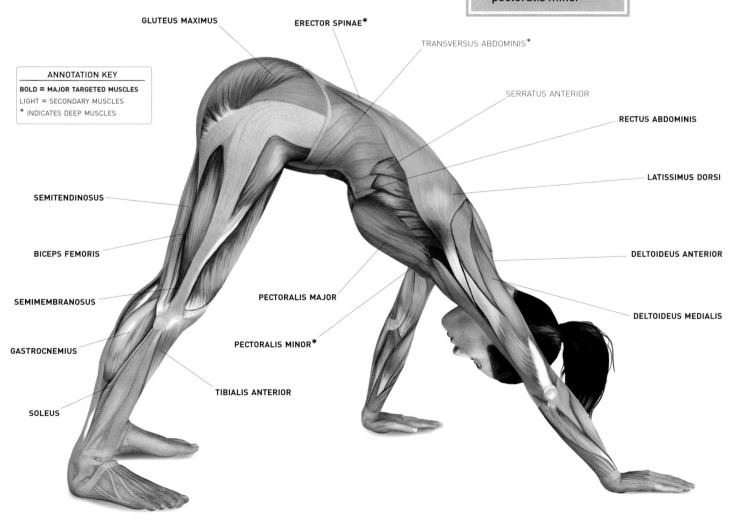

GLUTEUS MAXIMUS

ERECTOR SPINAE*

TRANSVERSUS ABDOMINIS*

SERRATUS ANTERIOR

RECTUS ABDOMINIS

LATISSIMUS DORSI

DELTOIDEUS ANTERIOR

DELTOIDEUS MEDIALIS

SEMITENDINOSUS

BICEPS FEMORIS

SEMIMEMBRANOSUS

GASTROCNEMIUS

SOLEUS

TIBIALIS ANTERIOR

PECTORALIS MINOR*

PECTORALIS MAJOR

WORKOUT B

All-Around Challenge

Start your joint health regimen at the top, with a workout that targets your neck and shoulders. Whether you spend hours at your desk peering at a computer screen or toss heavy weights like a book-laden backpack across your shoulders every day, this area can too often hold a lot of tension. Try this beginner-level workout to help counteract that tightness and keep your shoulder and neck joints moving smoothly.

1. ALTERNATING SIT-UP
(Pages 164–165)

Perform two sets, alternating sides for 15 repetitions on each side.

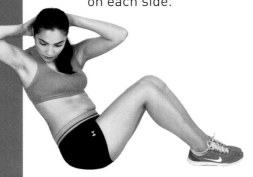

2. LEMON SQUEEZER
(Pages 166–167)

Perform 10 repetitions

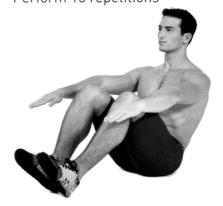

3. FOUR-COUNT OVERHEAD
(Pages 168–170)

Perform 10 repetitions.

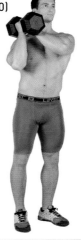

4. SHOULDER DRILL
(Pages 171–172)

Perform 10 repetitions.

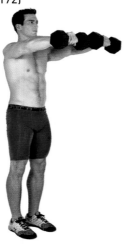

5. PUSH-UP WALKOUT
(Pages 173–174)

Perform 10 repetitions.

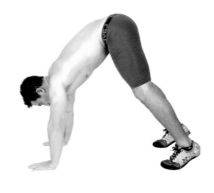

6. UP-DOWN
(Pages 175–176)

Perform for five minutes.

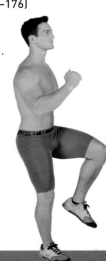

7. KNEE RAISE WITH LATERAL EXTENSION
(Pages 177–178)

Alternate sides for 10 to 12 repetitions on each side.

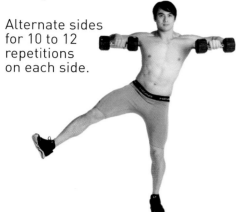

8. DIVER'S PUSH-UP
(Pages 179–180)

Perform 15 to 20 repetitions.

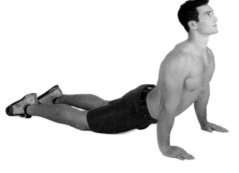

9. LATERAL-EXTENSION REVERSE LUNGE
(Pages 181–182)

Perform two sets, alternating sides for 10 repetitions on each side.

10. SWISS BALL BRIDGE
(Pages 183–184)

Perform 10 to 15 repetitions.

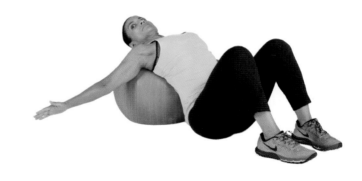

11. SWISS BALL PIKE
(Pages 185–186)

Perform 10 repetitions.

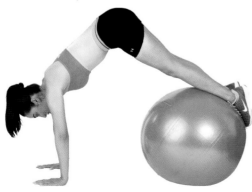

12. BACKWARD BALL STRETCH
(Pages 187–188)

Perform one repetitions.

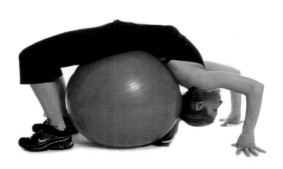

ALTERNATING SIT-UP

1 Lie faceup on a mat with your legs slightly bent and your hands behind your head.

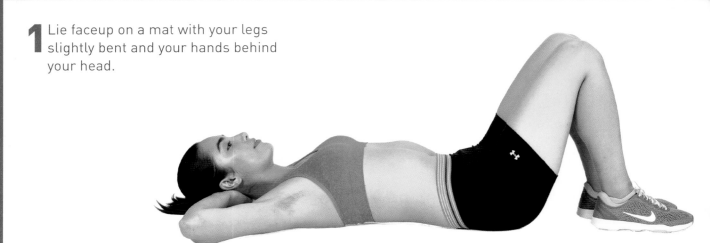

2 Begin to lift your upper back from the mat

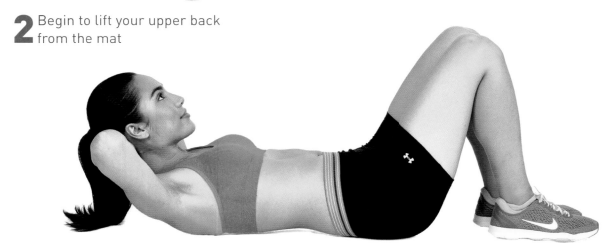

3 Push through your heels for support and raise your trunk off the mat.

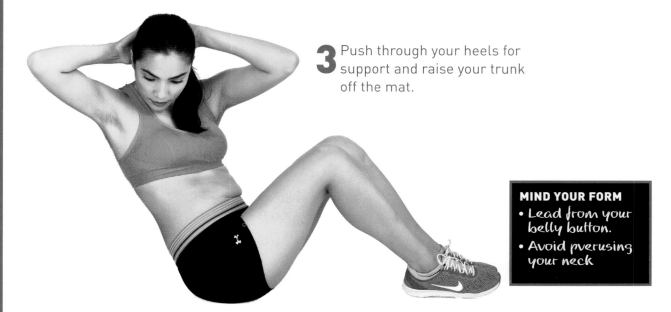

MIND YOUR FORM
- Lead from your belly button.
- Avoid overusing your neck

3 Rotate to the left so your elbow touches your opposite knee, and contract your abdominals.

4 Lower and repeat, rotating to the other side. Continue to alternate sides for 15 repetitions per side.

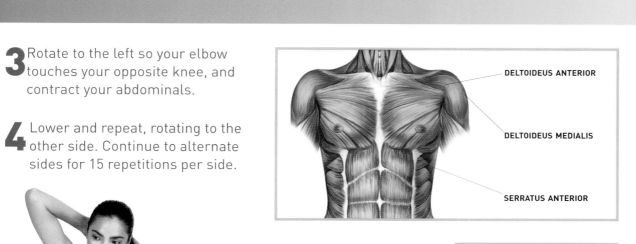

DELTOIDEUS ANTERIOR

DELTOIDEUS MEDIALIS

SERRATUS ANTERIOR

MAJOR TARGETED MUSCLES

- rectus abdominis
- erector spinae
- deltoideus posterior
- serratus anterior
- deltoideus anterior
- deltoideus medialis
- obliquus externus
- obliquus internus

ANNOTATION KEY

BOLD = MAJOR TARGETED MUSCLES
LIGHT = SECONDARY MUSCLES
* INDICATES DEEP MUSCLES

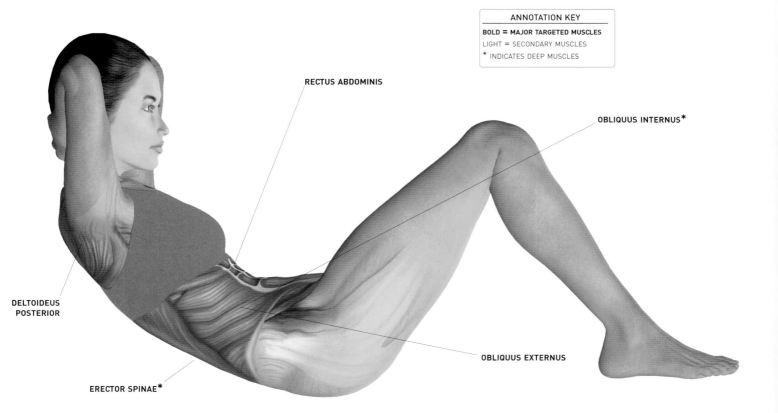

RECTUS ABDOMINIS

OBLIQUUS INTERNUS*

DELTOIDEUS POSTERIOR

OBLIQUUS EXTERNUS

ERECTOR SPINAE*

LEMON SQUEEZER

1 Lie supine on a mat with your arms flat by your side.

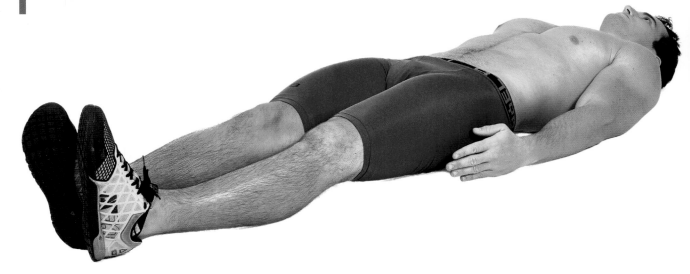

2 Lift your legs, head, neck, and shoulders slightly off the floor, being careful not to arch your lower back. Your arms should be raised and parallel to the floor.

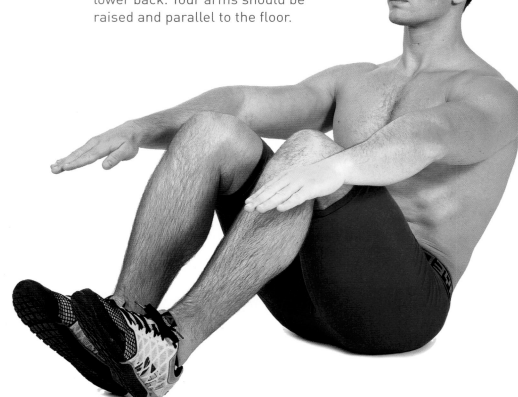

MIND YOUR FORM
- Keep your chin tucked and your thigh muscles firm throughout the exercise.
- Avoid allowing your shoulders to lift up toward your ears.

3 Pause at the top of the movement, and then lower yourself almost to the starting position. Repeat the motion without completely lying down on the mat. Perform two set of 15 times repetitions.

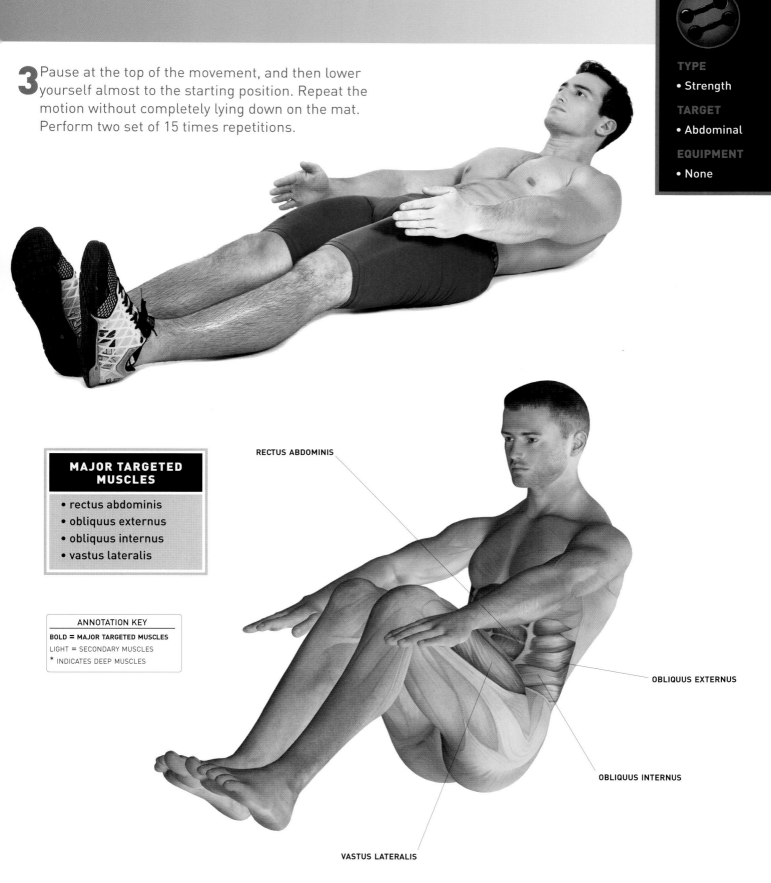

MAJOR TARGETED MUSCLES

• rectus abdominis
• obliquus externus
• obliquus internus
• vastus lateralis

ANNOTATION KEY

BOLD = MAJOR TARGETED MUSCLES
LIGHT = SECONDARY MUSCLES
* INDICATES DEEP MUSCLES

RECTUS ABDOMINIS

OBLIQUUS EXTERNUS

OBLIQUUS INTERNUS

VASTUS LATERALIS

FOUR-COUNT OVERHEAD

1 Stand with your feet hip-width apart. With both hands, grasp a dumbbell of any weight you can press overhead, and bring it to your right shoulder. This is your starting position.

2 Press the weight overhead with your arms straight and steady for count 1.

3 Lower the weight to your left shoulder for count 2.

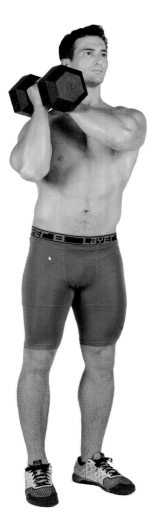

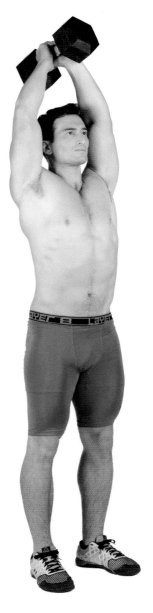

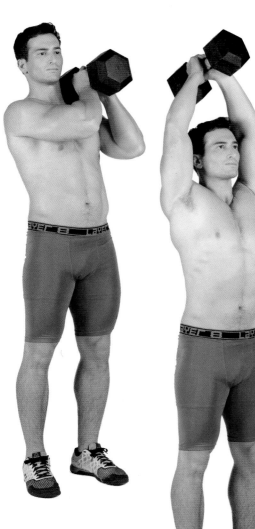

4 Press the weight overhead with your arms straight for 3.

MIND YOUR FORM
- Keep your glutes and abdominals tight.
- Maintain and steady beat, moving quickly but with control.

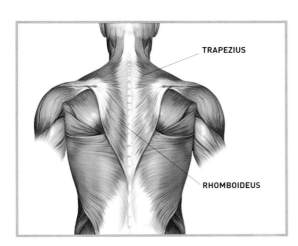

TRAPEZIUS

RHOMBOIDEUS

TYPE
• Strength
• Cardio

TARGET
• Shoulders

EQUIPMENT
• Dumbbells

5 Lower the weight to your right shoulder for count 4. Each time the weight touches your right shoulder equals one repetition. Each 1-to-4 count equals one repetition. Perform 10 repetitions to a 4-count rhthym

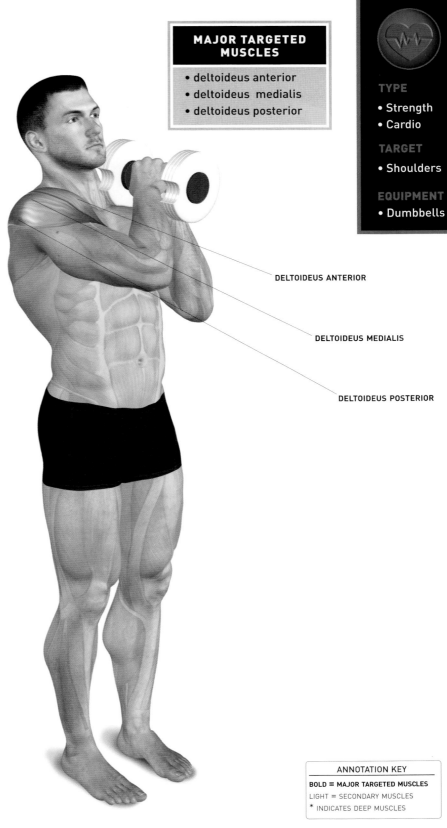

DELTOIDEUS ANTERIOR

DELTOIDEUS MEDIALIS

DELTOIDEUS POSTERIOR

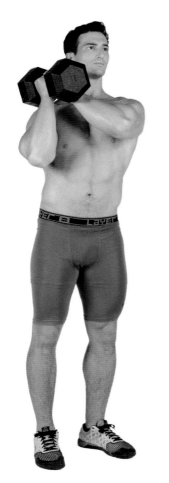

ANNOTATION KEY

BOLD = MAJOR TARGETED MUSCLES
LIGHT = SECONDARY MUSCLES
* INDICATES DEEP MUSCLES

SHOULDER DRILL

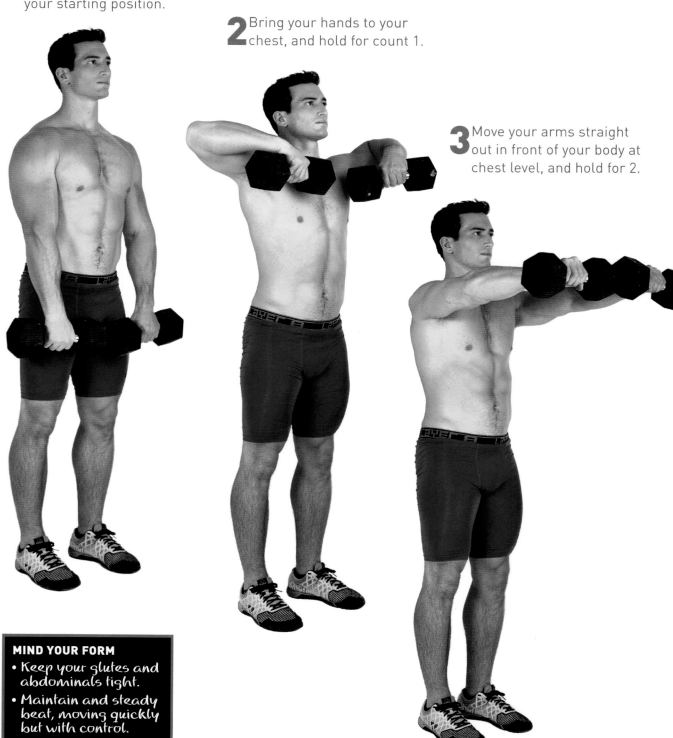

1 Stand with a dumbbell in each hand resting at the front of your thighs. This is your starting position.

2 Bring your hands to your chest, and hold for count 1.

3 Move your arms straight out in front of your body at chest level, and hold for 2.

MIND YOUR FORM
- Keep your glutes and abdominals tight.
- Maintain and steady beat, moving quickly but with control.

170

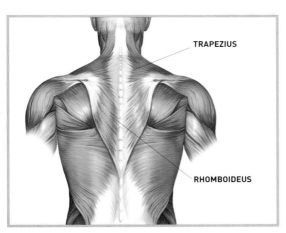

TRAPEZIUS

RHOMBOIDEUS

4 Bring your hands back to your chest, and hold for count 4.

5 Drop your arms to the front of each thigh for count 4. Each time your hands hit your thighs equals one rep. Perform 10 repetitions.

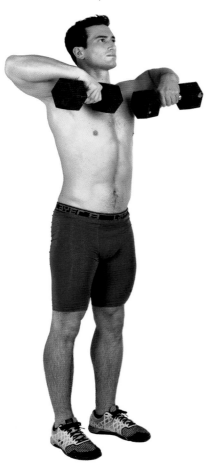

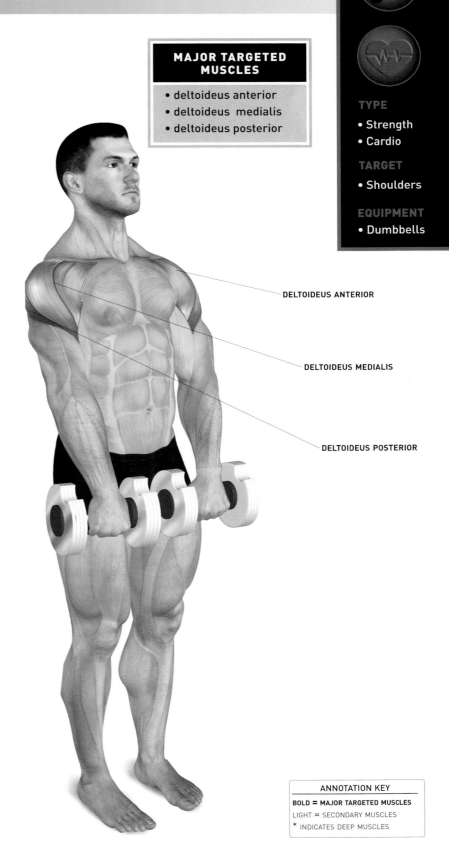

DELTOIDEUS ANTERIOR

DELTOIDEUS MEDIALIS

DELTOIDEUS POSTERIOR

PUSH-UP WALKOUT

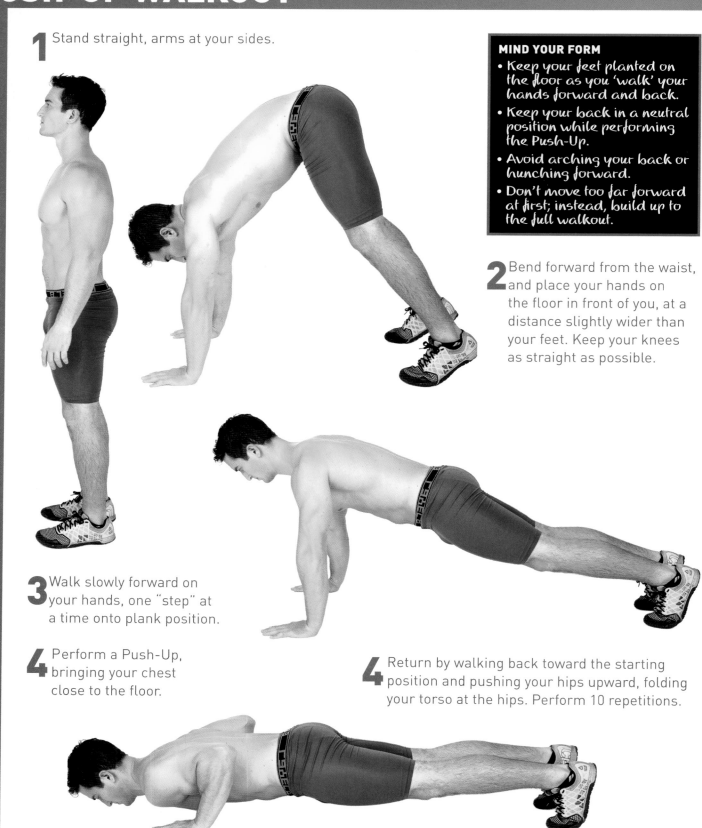

1 Stand straight, arms at your sides.

MIND YOUR FORM
- Keep your feet planted on the floor as you 'walk' your hands forward and back.
- Keep your back in a neutral position while performing the Push-Up.
- Avoid arching your back or hunching forward.
- Don't move too far forward at first; instead, build up to the full walkout.

2 Bend forward from the waist, and place your hands on the floor in front of you, at a distance slightly wider than your feet. Keep your knees as straight as possible.

3 Walk slowly forward on your hands, one "step" at a time onto plank position.

4 Perform a Push-Up, bringing your chest close to the floor.

4 Return by walking back toward the starting position and pushing your hips upward, folding your torso at the hips. Perform 10 repetitions.

172

TYPE
• Strength
TARGET
• Full body
EQUIPMENT
• None

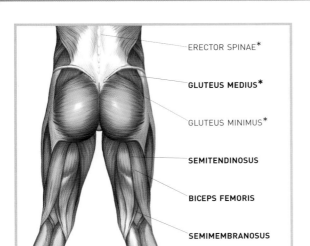

ERECTOR SPINAE*

GLUTEUS MEDIUS*

GLUTEUS MINIMUS*

SEMITENDINOSUS

BICEPS FEMORIS

SEMIMEMBRANOSUS

ANNOTATION KEY

BOLD = MAJOR SUPPORTING MUSCLES
LIGHT = SECONDARY MUSCLES
ITALIC = TENDONS & LIGAMENTS
* INDICATES DEEP MUSCLES

MAJOR TARGETED MUSCLES

- gluteus medius
- quadratus lumborum
- erector spinae
- latissimus dorsi
- trapezius
- pectoralis malor
- biceps femoris
- semitendinosus
- semimembranosus
- rectus abdominis
- coracobrachialis
- brachialis

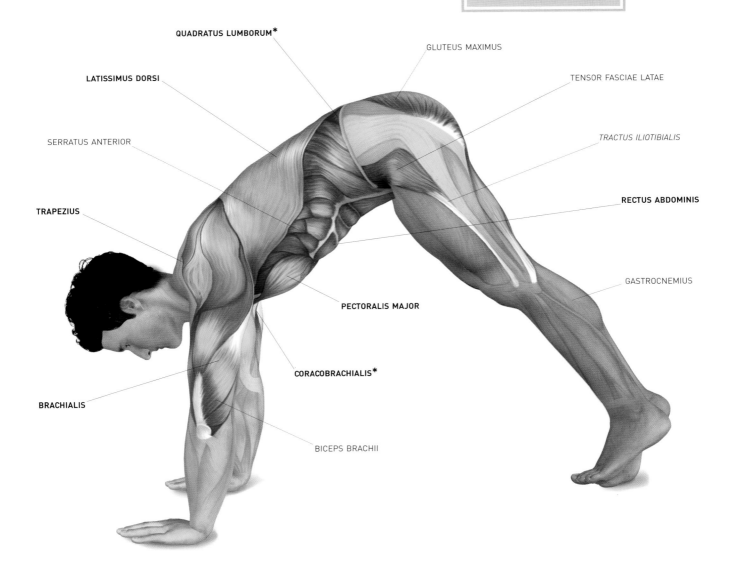

QUADRATUS LUMBORUM*

GLUTEUS MAXIMUS

LATISSIMUS DORSI

TENSOR FASCIAE LATAE

SERRATUS ANTERIOR

TRACTUS ILIOTIBIALIS

RECTUS ABDOMINIS

TRAPEZIUS

GASTROCNEMIUS

PECTORALIS MAJOR

BRACHIALIS

CORACOBRACHIALIS*

BICEPS BRACHII

UP-DOWN

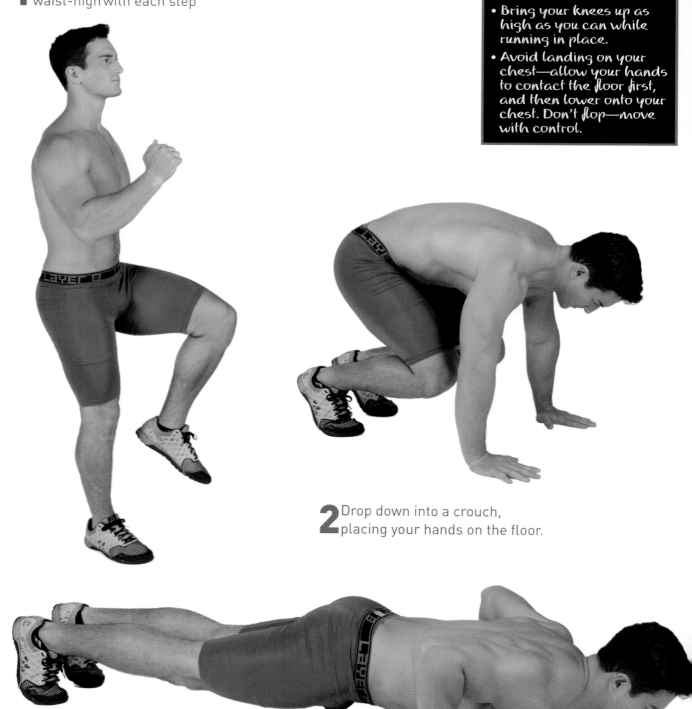

1 Run in place, bringing your knees waist-high with each step

MIND YOUR FORM
- Bring your knees up as high as you can while running in place.
- Avoid landing on your chest—allow your hands to contact the floor first, and then lower onto your chest. Don't flop—move with control.

2 Drop down into a crouch, placing your hands on the floor.

3 Kick your legs back, and touch your chest to the floor.

4 Immediately stand back up, and resume running with high knees as quickly as possible. Perform entire sequence as many times as you can in five minutes.

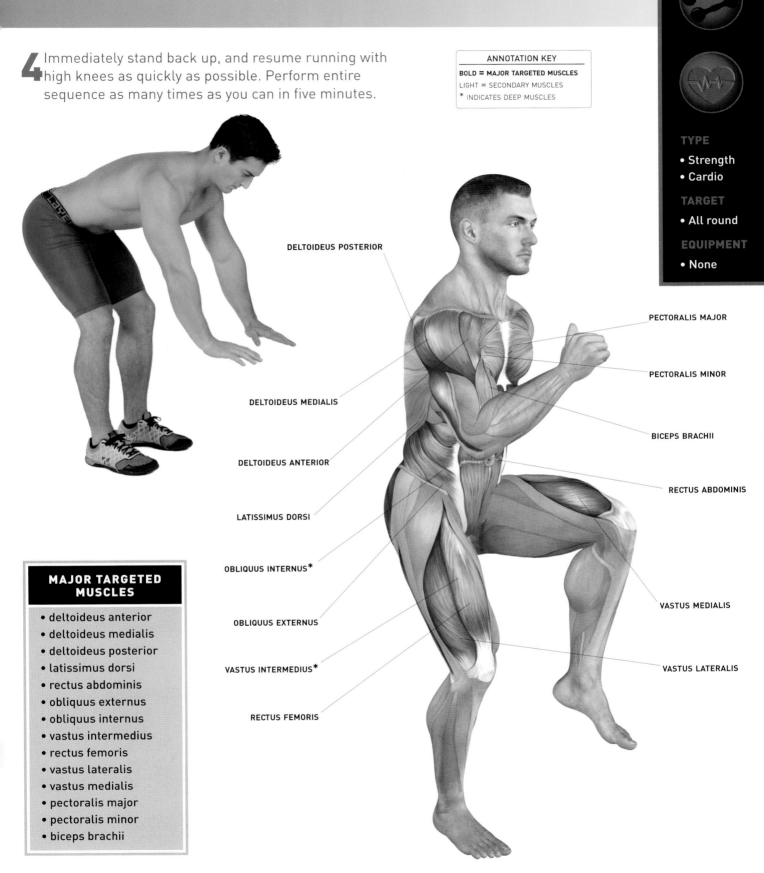

ANNOTATION KEY

BOLD = MAJOR TARGETED MUSCLES
LIGHT = SECONDARY MUSCLES
* INDICATES DEEP MUSCLES

TYPE
- Strength
- Cardio

TARGET
- All round

EQUIPMENT
- None

DELTOIDEUS POSTERIOR

DELTOIDEUS MEDIALIS

DELTOIDEUS ANTERIOR

LATISSIMUS DORSI

OBLIQUUS INTERNUS*

OBLIQUUS EXTERNUS

VASTUS INTERMEDIUS*

RECTUS FEMORIS

PECTORALIS MAJOR

PECTORALIS MINOR

BICEPS BRACHII

RECTUS ABDOMINIS

VASTUS MEDIALIS

VASTUS LATERALIS

MAJOR TARGETED MUSCLES

- deltoideus anterior
- deltoideus medialis
- deltoideus posterior
- latissimus dorsi
- rectus abdominis
- obliquus externus
- obliquus internus
- vastus intermedius
- rectus femoris
- vastus lateralis
- vastus medialis
- pectoralis major
- pectoralis minor
- biceps brachii

KNEE RAISE WITH LATERAL EXTENSION

1 Stand with your feet hip-width apart and your arms at your sides, a dumbbell in each hand.

2 Shifting your weight onto your left leg, bend your right knee, and raise your leg. At the same time, raise your arms until the weights are slightly below shoulder height. Take a moment or two to find your balance.

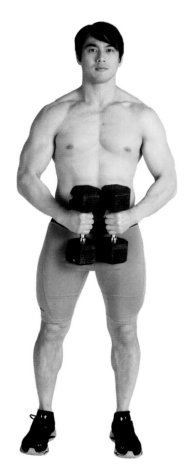

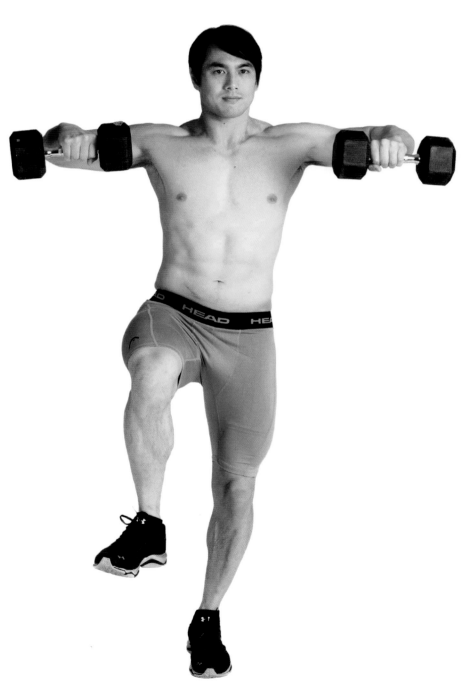

MIND YOUR FORM
- Keep your torso facing forward.
- Pull your navel toward your spine, and engage your abdominal muscles.
- Gaze forward.
- Maintain a neutral S-curve in your spine.
- Anchor your standing leg to the floor.
- Avoid twisting your torso to either side.

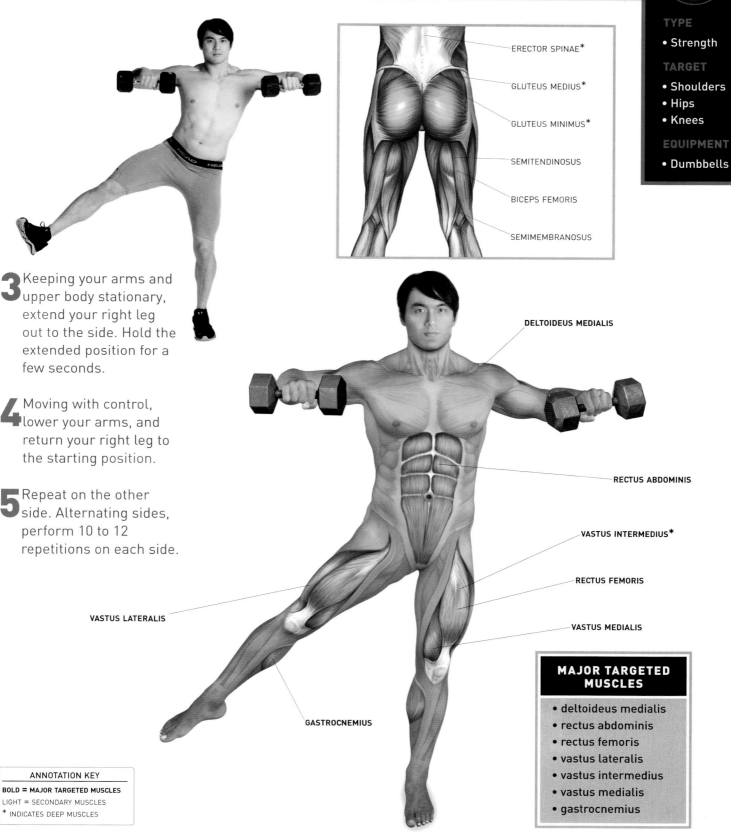

TYPE
• Strength

TARGET
• Shoulders
• Hips
• Knees

EQUIPMENT
• Dumbbells

ERECTOR SPINAE*

GLUTEUS MEDIUS*

GLUTEUS MINIMUS*

SEMITENDINOSUS

BICEPS FEMORIS

SEMIMEMBRANOSUS

3 Keeping your arms and upper body stationary, extend your right leg out to the side. Hold the extended position for a few seconds.

4 Moving with control, lower your arms, and return your right leg to the starting position.

5 Repeat on the other side. Alternating sides, perform 10 to 12 repetitions on each side.

DELTOIDEUS MEDIALIS

RECTUS ABDOMINIS

VASTUS INTERMEDIUS*

RECTUS FEMORIS

VASTUS LATERALIS

VASTUS MEDIALIS

GASTROCNEMIUS

MAJOR TARGETED MUSCLES

• deltoideus medialis
• rectus abdominis
• rectus femoris
• vastus lateralis
• vastus intermedius
• vastus medialis
• gastrocnemius

ANNOTATION KEY

BOLD = MAJOR TARGETED MUSCLES
LIGHT = SECONDARY MUSCLES
* INDICATES DEEP MUSCLES

DIVER'S PUSH-UP

1 Begin in a plank position with your hands on the floor in front of you. Push your hips upward so that your body forms an inverted V.

MIND YOUR FORM
- Position your arms firmly on the floor, securely grounding your fingers.
- Avoid letting your thighs or knees rest on the floor.

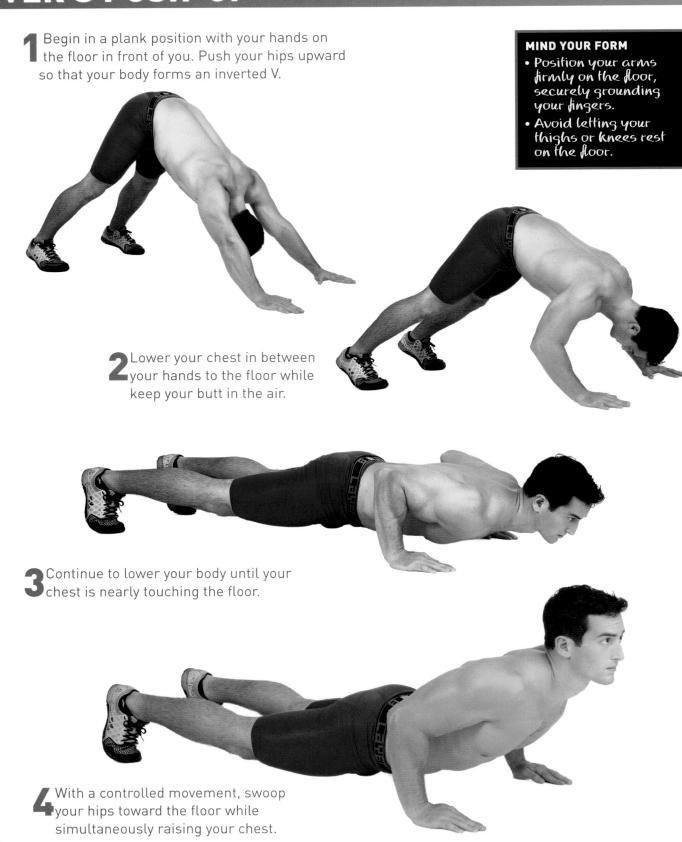

2 Lower your chest in between your hands to the floor while keep your butt in the air.

3 Continue to lower your body until your chest is nearly touching the floor.

4 With a controlled movement, swoop your hips toward the floor while simultaneously raising your chest.

5 Continue rising upward until you're looking toward the ceiling and your back is arched.

6 Swoop back down, and the repeat the entire sequence for 15 to 20 repetitions.

TYPE
- Strength
- Cardio

TARGET
- Full body

EQUIPMENT
- Mat

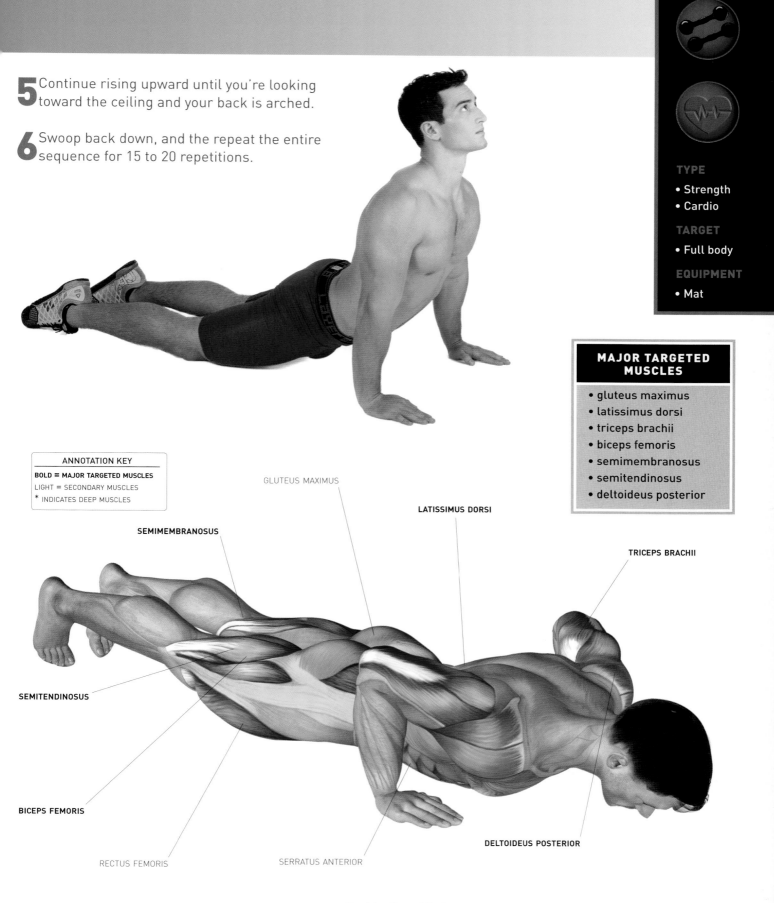

MAJOR TARGETED MUSCLES
- gluteus maximus
- latissimus dorsi
- triceps brachii
- biceps femoris
- semimembranosus
- semitendinosus
- deltoideus posterior

ANNOTATION KEY
BOLD = MAJOR TARGETED MUSCLES
LIGHT = SECONDARY MUSCLES
* INDICATES DEEP MUSCLES

GLUTEUS MAXIMUS

LATISSIMUS DORSI

SEMIMEMBRANOSUS

TRICEPS BRACHII

SEMITENDINOSUS

BICEPS FEMORIS

RECTUS FEMORIS

SERRATUS ANTERIOR

DELTOIDEUS POSTERIOR

LATERAL-EXTENSION REVERSE LUNGE

1 Stand with your feet hip-width apart and your arms at your sides, a dumbbell in each hand.

2 Take a big step backward with your right foot, bending your knees as you do so. As you lower your body, flexing your left knee and hip until your right leg is almost in contact with the floor, simultaneously raise your arms to the side until they are level with your shoulders.

3 When your front thigh is roughly parallel to the floor, push through your left heel, and bring your right foot forward to meet your left. At the same time, bring the dumbbells back to your sides to return to the starting position.

4 Switch legs, and repeat on the other side, and then continue to alternate sides for a total of 10 repetitions on each leg. Perform two sets.

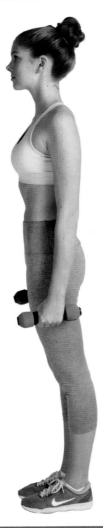

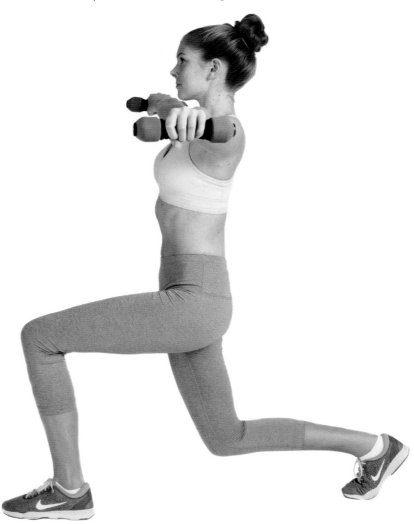

MIND YOUR FORM
- Keep your shoulders pressed downward.
- Keep your neck relaxed.
- Maintain upright form in your upper body as you lower and then raise your body.
- Avoid twisting either hip.
- Avoid hunching or tensing your shoulders.
- Avoid arching your back or hunching forward.

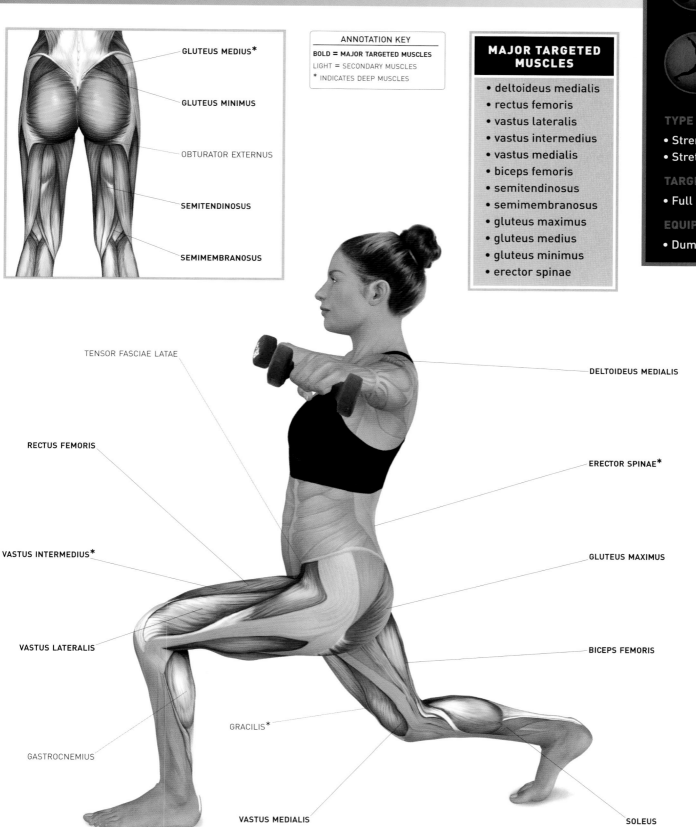

GLUTEUS MEDIUS*

GLUTEUS MINIMUS

OBTURATOR EXTERNUS

SEMITENDINOSUS

SEMIMEMBRANOSUS

ANNOTATION KEY

BOLD = MAJOR TARGETED MUSCLES
LIGHT = SECONDARY MUSCLES
* INDICATES DEEP MUSCLES

MAJOR TARGETED MUSCLES

- deltoideus medialis
- rectus femoris
- vastus lateralis
- vastus intermedius
- vastus medialis
- biceps femoris
- semitendinosus
- semimembranosus
- gluteus maximus
- gluteus medius
- gluteus minimus
- erector spinae

TYPE
- Strength
- Stretch

TARGET
- Full body

EQUIPMENT
- Dumbbells

TENSOR FASCIAE LATAE

RECTUS FEMORIS

VASTUS INTERMEDIUS*

VASTUS LATERALIS

GRACILIS*

GASTROCNEMIUS

VASTUS MEDIALIS

DELTOIDEUS MEDIALIS

ERECTOR SPINAE*

GLUTEUS MAXIMUS

BICEPS FEMORIS

SOLEUS

SWISS BALL BRIDGE

1 Sit on the floor with your back against a Swiss ball. Bend your knees to 90 degrees and spread your arms wide at shoulder height.

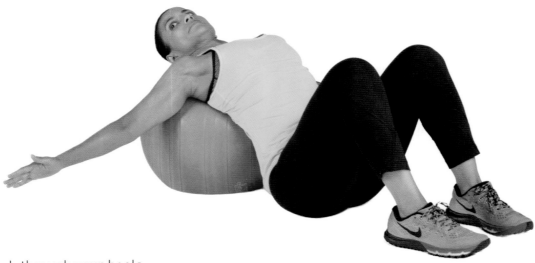

2 Push through your heels, and, using your glutes and hamstrings, raise your hips upward as you roll your back up the ball until your torso is aligned with your thighs.

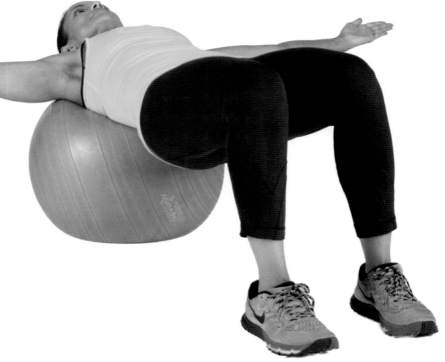

MIND YOUR FORM
- Contract your glutes and hold your stomach tight to keep your hips and shoulders parallel to the floor.
- To maintain your upper-body form, you can hold a pole or broomstick with your arms outspread.

182

3 Hold for 10 seconds, and then lower yourself back down. Peform 10 to 15 repetitions.

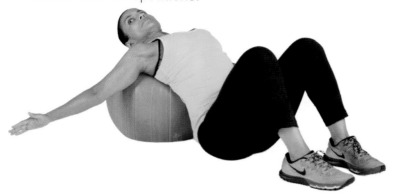

MAJOR TARGETED MUSCLES

- rectus abdominis
- transversus abdominis
- obliquus externus
- obliquus internus
- rectus femoris
- vastus lateralis
- vastus intermedius
- vastus medialis

TYPE
- Strength

TARGET
- Abdominals
- Thighs

EQUIPMENT
- Swiss ball

ANNOTATION KEY

BOLD = MAJOR TARGETED MUSCLES
LIGHT = SECONDARY MUSCLES
* INDICATES DEEP MUSCLES

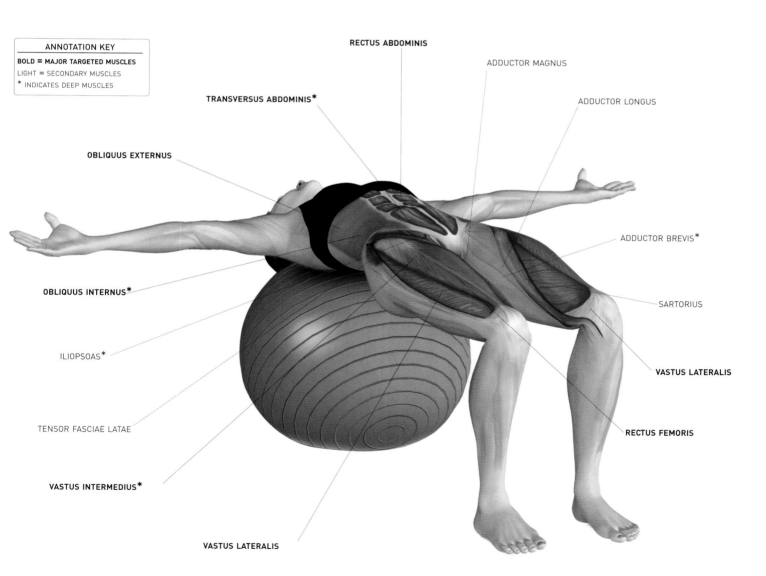

RECTUS ABDOMINIS

ADDUCTOR MAGNUS

TRANSVERSUS ABDOMINIS*

ADDUCTOR LONGUS

OBLIQUUS EXTERNUS

ADDUCTOR BREVIS*

OBLIQUUS INTERNUS*

SARTORIUS

ILIOPSOAS*

VASTUS LATERALIS

TENSOR FASCIAE LATAE

RECTUS FEMORIS

VASTUS INTERMEDIUS*

VASTUS LATERALIS

SWISS BALL PIKE

1 Kneel on your hands and knees with hands, and prop your feet on top of a Swiss ball.

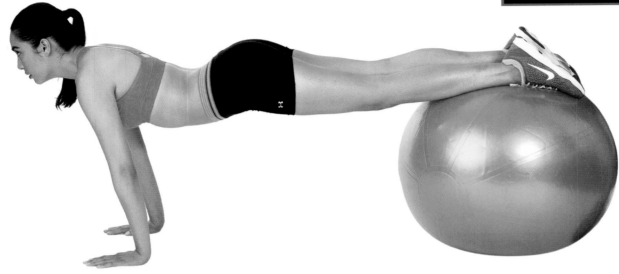

2 While keeping your legs straight, roll the ball toward your body while raising your hips as high as you are able. Lower, and repeat for 10 repetitions.

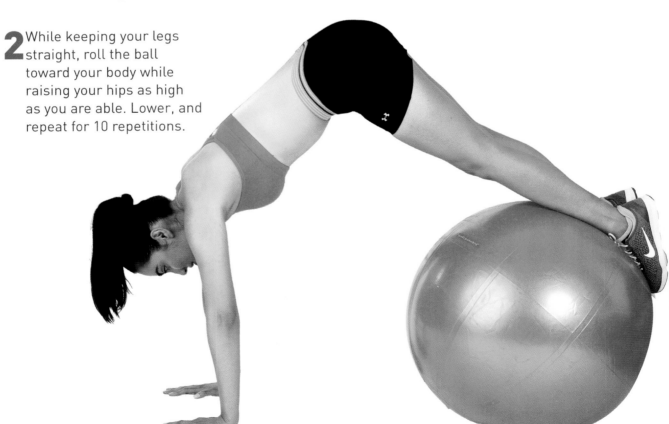

MAJOR TARGETED MUSCLES

- iliopsoas
- tensor fasciae latae
- vastus medialis
- sartorius
- erector spinae
- obliquus externus
- latissimus dorsi
- trapezius
- deltoideus anterior
- serratus anterior
- pectoralis major
- pectoralis minor
- coracobrachialis
- triceps brachii
- extensor digitorum
- quadratus lumborum
- vastus lateralis
- rectus femoris

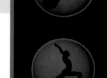

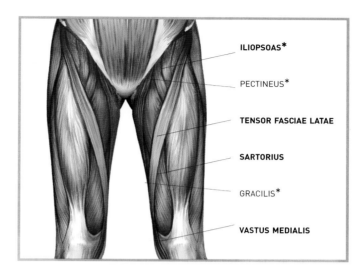

ILIOPSOAS*

PECTINEUS*

TENSOR FASCIAE LATAE

SARTORIUS

GRACILIS*

VASTUS MEDIALIS

TYPE
- Strength
- Stretch

TARGET
- Full body

EQUIPMENT
- Swiss ball

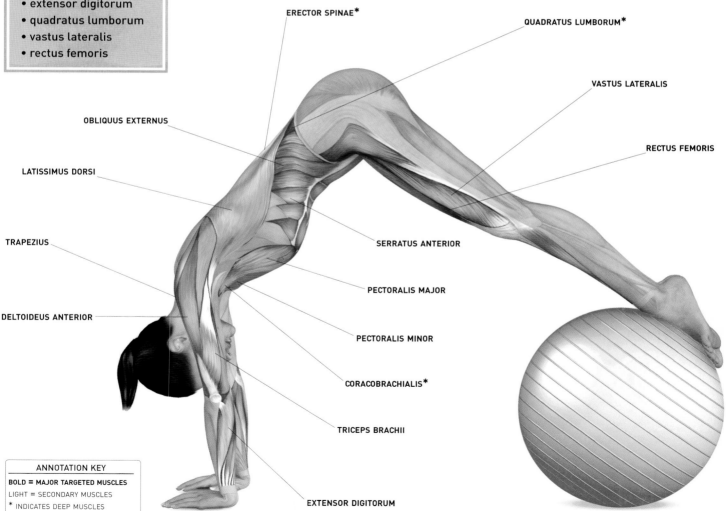

ERECTOR SPINAE*

QUADRATUS LUMBORUM*

VASTUS LATERALIS

OBLIQUUS EXTERNUS

RECTUS FEMORIS

LATISSIMUS DORSI

SERRATUS ANTERIOR

TRAPEZIUS

PECTORALIS MAJOR

DELTOIDEUS ANTERIOR

PECTORALIS MINOR

CORACOBRACHIALIS*

TRICEPS BRACHII

EXTENSOR DIGITORUM

ANNOTATION KEY

BOLD = MAJOR TARGETED MUSCLES
LIGHT = SECONDARY MUSCLES
* INDICATES DEEP MUSCLES

BACKWARD BALL STRETCH

1 Sit on a Swiss ball in a well-balanced, neutral position, with your hips directly over the center of the ball.

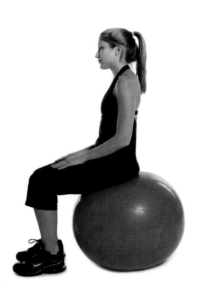

2 Raise your arms while maintaining good balance, and begin to extend them behind you.

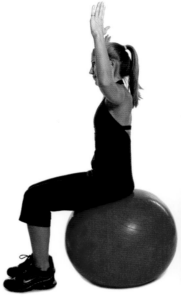

> **MIND YOUR FORM**
> - Maintain good balance throughout the stretch.
> - Move slowly and with control.
> - Keep your head on the ball until you have dropped your knees all the way down as you release from the stretch.
> - Don't allow the ball to shift to the side.
> - Avoid holding the extended position for too long, or until you feel dizzy.

3 As you continue to extend your hands backward, walk your feet forward, allowing the ball to roll up your spine.

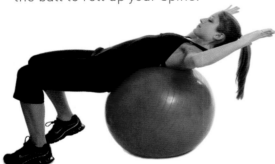

4 As your hands touch the floor, extend your legs as far forward as you comfortably can. Hold this position for 10 seconds.

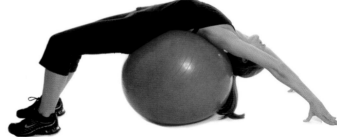

5 To deepen the stretch, extend your arms, and walk your legs and hands closer to the ball. Hold this position for 10 seconds.

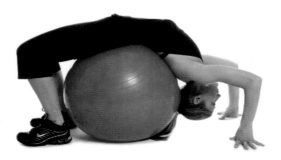

6 To release the stretch, bend your knees, drop your hips to the floor, lift your head off the ball, and then walk your feet back to the starting position.

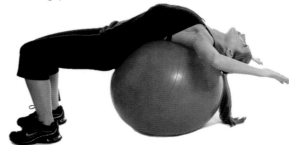

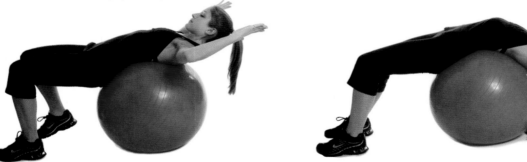

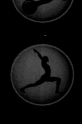

MAJOR TARGETED MUSCLES

- deltoideus medialis
- iliopsoas
- latissimus dorsi
- serratus anterior
- pectoralis major
- pectoralis minor
- ligamentum longitudinale anterius

ANNOTATION KEY

BOLD = MAJOR TARGETED MUSCLES
LIGHT = SECONDARY MUSCLES
ITALIC = *TENDONS & LIGAMENTS*
* INDICATES DEEP MUSCLES

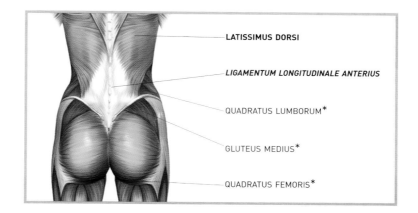

LATISSIMUS DORSI

LIGAMENTUM LONGITUDINALE ANTERIUS

QUADRATUS LUMBORUM*

GLUTEUS MEDIUS*

QUADRATUS FEMORIS*

TYPE
- Strength
- Stretch

TARGET
- Full body

EQUIPMENT
- Swiss ball

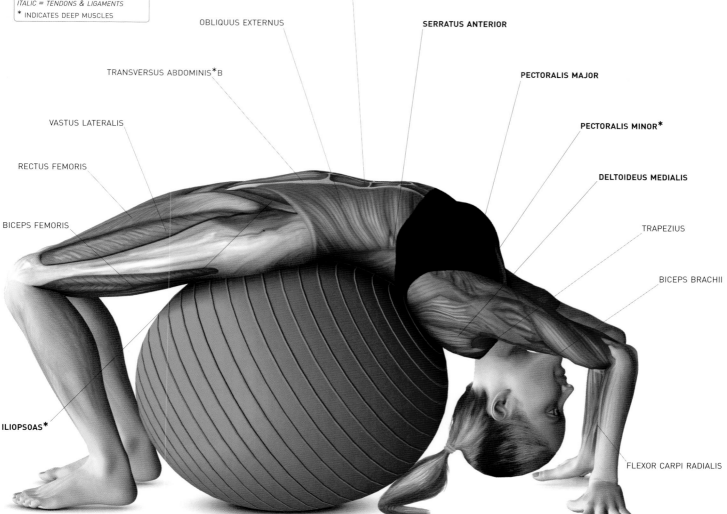

RECTUS ABDOMINIS

OBLIQUUS EXTERNUS

TRANSVERSUS ABDOMINIS*B

VASTUS LATERALIS

RECTUS FEMORIS

BICEPS FEMORIS

ILIOPSOAS*

SERRATUS ANTERIOR

PECTORALIS MAJOR

PECTORALIS MINOR*

DELTOIDEUS MEDIALIS

TRAPEZIUS

BICEPS BRACHII

FLEXOR CARPI RADIALIS

INDEX OF EXERCISES

A re you looking for a particular exercise? Use this handy visual guide to find the one you need. You can also use this index to craft your own personlized Healthy Hearts workout.

ALTERNATING SIT-UP
(Pages 164–165)

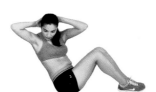

BACKWARD BALL STRETCH
(Pages 186–187)

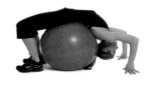

BEAR CRAWL
(Pages 98–99)

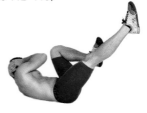

BICYCLE CRUNCH
(Pages 112–113)

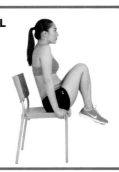

BOTTOMS-UP KETTLEBELL CLEAN
(Pages 156–157)

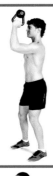

BURPEE
(Pages 118–119)

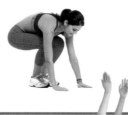

BUTT KICK
(Pages 60–61)

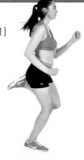

CHAIR ABDOMINAL CRUNCH
(Pages 50–51)

CHAIR PLIÉ
(Pages 32–32)

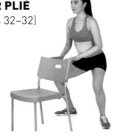

CHAIR POSE
(Pages 40– 41)

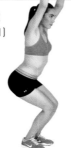

CHAIR SQUAT
(Pages 30–31)

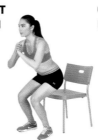

CLAMSHELL SERIES
(Pages 114–115)

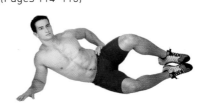

CROSSOVER STEP-UP
(Pages 100–101)

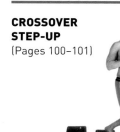

CURLING STEP-AND-RAISE
(Pages 56–57)

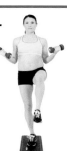

DIAGONAL REACH
(Pages 72–73)

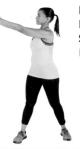

DOUBLE KETTLEBELL SNATCH
(Pages 158–159)

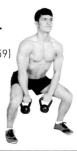

DIVER'S PUSH-UP
(Pages 178–179)

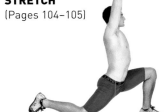

FOUR-COUNT OVERHEAD
(Pages 168–169)

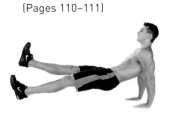

FRONT PLANK WITH LEG LIFT
(Pages 110–111)

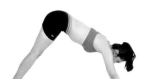

HIGH KNEES
(Pages 48–49)

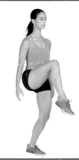

HIP-TO THIGH STRETCH
(Pages 104–105)

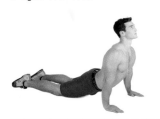

ILIOTIBIAL BAND STRETCH
(Pages 74–75)

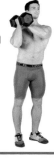

INCHWORM
(Pages 160–161)

INVERTED LEG EXTENSION
(Pages 126–127)

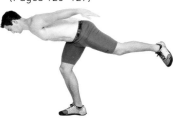

KNEE RAISE WITH LATERAL EXTENSION
(Pages 176–177)

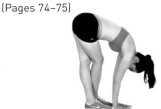

LATERAL BOUNDING
(Pages 86–87)

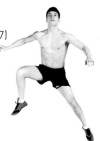

LATERAL-EXTENSION LATERAL LUNGE
(Pages 44–45)

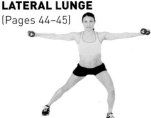

LATERAL-EXTENSION REVERSE LUNGE
(Pages 180–181)

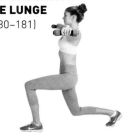

LATERAL LUNGE
(Pages 42–43)

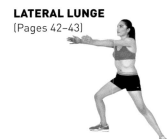

LATERAL STEP-AND-CURL
(Pages 36–37)

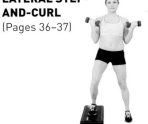

LATERAL STEP-DOWN
(Pages 58–59)

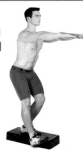

LATERAL STEP-OVER
(Pages 128–129)

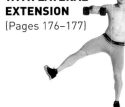

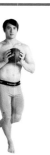

INDEX OF EXERCISES

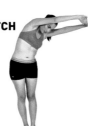
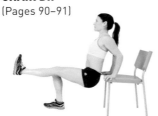
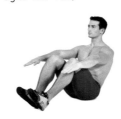
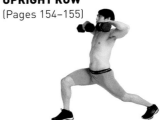
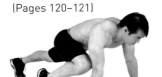
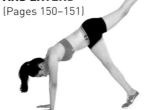
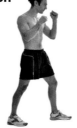
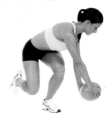
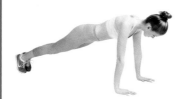
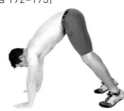
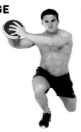
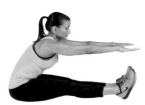
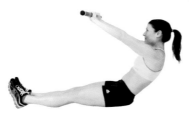
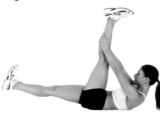
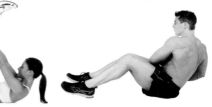
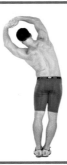
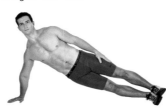
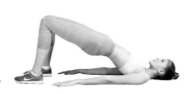
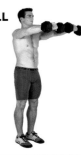

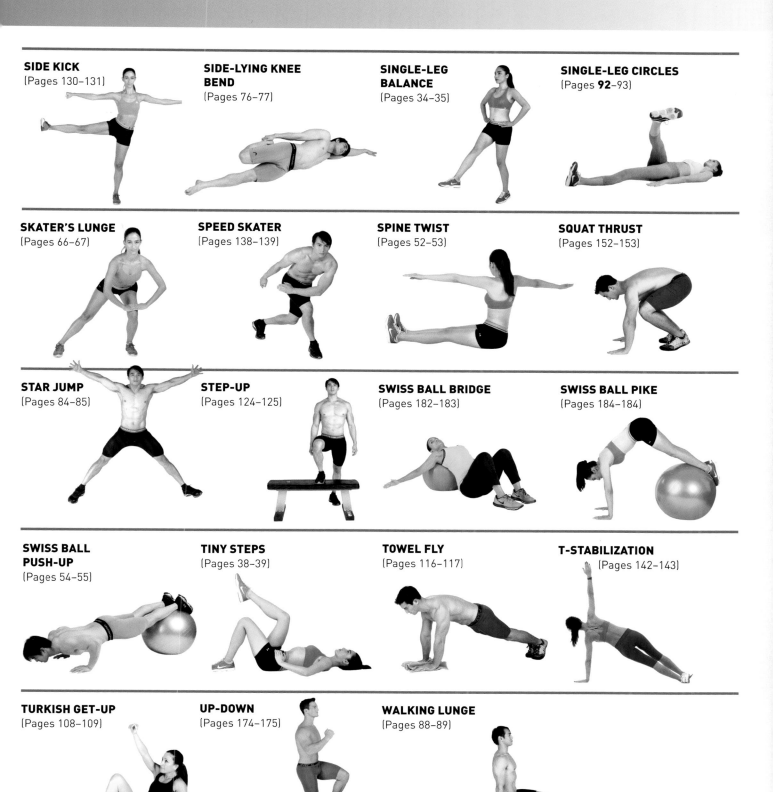

SIDE KICK
(Pages 130–131)

SIDE-LYING KNEE BEND
(Pages 76–77)

SINGLE-LEG BALANCE
(Pages 34–35)

SINGLE-LEG CIRCLES
(Pages **92**–93)

SKATER'S LUNGE
(Pages 66–67)

SPEED SKATER
(Pages 138–139)

SPINE TWIST
(Pages 52–53)

SQUAT THRUST
(Pages 152–153)

STAR JUMP
(Pages 84–85)

STEP-UP
(Pages 124–125)

SWISS BALL BRIDGE
(Pages 182–183)

SWISS BALL PIKE
(Pages 184–184)

SWISS BALL PUSH-UP
(Pages 54–55)

TINY STEPS
(Pages 38–39)

TOWEL FLY
(Pages 116–117)

T-STABILIZATION
(Pages 142–143)

TURKISH GET-UP
(Pages 108–109)

UP-DOWN
(Pages 174–175)

WALKING LUNGE
(Pages 88–89)

CREDITS AND ACKNOWLEDGMENTS

Illustration Credits
All anatomical illustrations by Hector Diaz/3DLabz Animation Limited
Insets by Linda Bucklin/Shutterstock.com

Photography Credits
ALL PHOTOS BY NAILA RUECHEL
with the following exceptions:

JONATHAN CONKLIN PHOTOGRAPHY
page 82, 102, 108–109, 110, 144, 186

FINE ARTS PHOTOGRAPHY GROUP
page 36, 44, 56,90, 94, 96, 146, 158

The following images courtesy Shutterstock.com

page 10 viagraphix.net; 11 Rocketclips, Inc.; 12,18 Africa Studio;
14–15 Jacob Lund; 16 marekuliasz; 17 frenkel vic; 19 Anatolii Riepin;
20 Dragon Images; 21 David Tadevosian; 22 (left) Dmytro Zinkevych;
22 (right) jurgenfr; 23 Nicotombo; 26–27, 78–79, 134–135 Maridav;
118, 143 Mihai Blanaru;

Acknowledgments
*Moseley Road and photographer Naila Ruechel would like to thank
models Roya Carreras, Alex Geissbuehler, Caroline Harty, Natasha
Walker, and Philip Chan.*